Palgrave Studies in Science, Knowledge and Policy

Series Editors
Katherine Smith
University of Edinburgh
Edinburgh, United Kingdom

Richard Freeman
University of Edinburgh
Edinburgh, United Kingdom

Many of the questions which concern us in our social, political and economic lives are questions of knowledge, whether they concern the extent and consequences of climate change, the efficacy of new drugs, the scope of surveillance technologies or the accreditation and performance of individuals and organizations. This is because what we know – how we acquire and apply knowledge of various kinds – shapes the ways in which problems are identified and understood; how laws, rules and norms are constructed and maintained, and which goods and services offered to whom. 'Who gets what, when, how', in Lasswell's phrase, depends very much on who knows what, when, how. In our personal, professional and public lives, knowledge is a key resource. It matters in policy not only as a guide to decision making but because, in many circumstances, to be knowledgeable is to be powerful. Some kinds of knowledge are created and held by small numbers of specialists, while others are widely distributed and quickly shared. The credibility and authority of different kinds of knowledge varies over time and our means of developing and sharing knowledge are currently undergoing rapid changes as new digital technologies and social media platforms emerge. This book series is an interdisciplinary forum to explore these issues and more. In short, we are interested in the politics of knowledge.

More information about this series at
http://www.springer.com/series/14592

John Boswell

The Real War on Obesity

Contesting Knowledge and Meaning in a Public Health Crisis

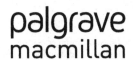

John Boswell
Politics and International Relations
University of Southampton
Southampton, United Kingdom

Palgrave Studies in Science, Knowledge and Policy
ISBN 978-1-349-84502-6   ISBN 978-1-137-58252-2   (eBook)
DOI 10.1057/978-1-137-58252-2

Library of Congress Control Number: 2016937726

Cover illustration: © HA Photos / Alamy Stock Photo

Printed on acid-free paper

This Palgrave Macmillan imprint is published by Springer Nature
The registered company is Macmillan Publishers Ltd. London

Acknowledgements

This book has taken a number of years to come to fruition and there are, naturally, a number of people to thank for helping me along the way. Top of the list are my wife Seahee and our boys Max, Toby, and Dominic. They have provided amazing support that has enabled me to pursue my interests, in the process moving our lives back and forth across the world a number of times. I am eternally grateful. I also thank my late grandfather for his tremendous help in a time of need, my parents for their unconditional faith in me throughout, my parents-in-law for their considerable patience, and my siblings for their interest and support.

Among my academic family, I thank Carolyn Hendriks first and foremost. Carolyn helped gently guide me through the initial project and put me on the way to an academic career. A number of other senior figures at the Australian National University (ANU) gave important advice along the way as well, but I reserve special mention for the thorough feedback John Dryzek was always willing to give and the good-humoured meetings that John Uhr would indulge of me. As important as the faculty were my fellow peers on the PhD journey. I thank especially Phil Baker, Lhawang Ugyel, Fiona Downs, Patrick Doupe, and Mary Milne for giving great feedback and being useful sounding boards as I worked my way through things. Again, special mention to two in particular though—Jack Corbett and Catherine Settle—who have become great friends and will hopefully remain long-time collaborators.

A number of colleagues at my new home in Southampton have provided useful advice as I have turned the thesis into a book. Rod Rhodes, David Owen, and Will Jennings have helped me to frame the book in a way that I think broadens its appeal and potential impact. I also thank the series editors, Kat Smith and Richard Freeman, for their useful feedback on my initial pitch, and for their support of my vision for the book. The publisher's anonymous readers have also provided enormously constructive feedback which has helped to sharpen the analysis in important ways.

On top of these academic colleagues it is also incumbent on me to thank my interview participants—all 45 of them—who were so instrumental in the success of the project. I thank them for their willingness to open up on this topic and share their deepest reflections. An abiding impression was how thoughtful so many of them were and how interested they were in the perspective I brought to the topic. I hope that they are able to enjoy, and perhaps even get something useful out of, the analysis that follows.

Along with the publisher, it is also important that I acknowledge the following for permission to reproduce excerpts from copyright material:

- Sage for Boswell, J forthcoming. 'The performance of political narratives: How Australia and Britain's "fat bombs" fizzled out', *British Journal of Political and International Relations*, pp. 1–17. DOI: 10.1177/1369148816630232.
- Taylor and Francis for Boswell, J 2015, 'Toxic narratives and the deliberative system: How the ghost of nanny stalks the obesity debate', *Policy Studies*, vol. 36, no. 3, pp. 314–328.
- Springer for Boswell, J 2014, '"Hoisted with our own petard': Evidence and democratic deliberation on obesity'. *Policy Sciences*, vol. 47, no. 4, pp. 345–365.

Finally, I thank Philippa Grand and Judith Allan at Palgrave for their editorial assistance.

Contents

List of Boxes

List of Tables

1

Introducing the *Real* 'War on Obesity'

Obesity is one of the most significant new challenges to have emerged for policymakers in the twenty-first century. Long considered a private matter, in recent times obesity has become associated with mounting concerns about costs to the health service and the wider economy. There is also a growing perception that societal factors, and not just individual failings, are responsible for this trend. And as a result obesity rose rapidly up the public agenda in the first decade of the century. What began as agitation within the health community (see WHO 2000) quickly spread to the political realm. By the mid- to late-2000s, it was an issue the authorities could not afford to ignore. In 2007, the much-hyped Foresight report highlighted the scale of the challenge facing the British government, and in particular sounded a dire warning about the consequences of inadequate action to address the obesity trend. A year later in Australia, the Preventative Health Task Force, similarly anticipated in public health circles, issued an equally stark assessment to the Commonwealth government. Obesity was, according to these experts and the political figures they mobilised, an 'epidemic', a 'tsunami', a 'time bomb'. And in response to this looming threat, the 'war on obesity' was born.

© The Editor(s) (if applicable) and The Author(s) 2016   1
J. Boswell, *The Real War on Obesity*,
DOI 10.1057/978-1-137-58252-2_1

Though obesity remains an issue of fitful attention for high politics, over half a decade later, it has, unmistakably, slipped down the public agenda. It no longer commands the same attention of Prime Ministers, health czars, celebrities, or editorial writers. Obesity is, in the choice words of one journalist interviewed for the project, 'just not sexy anymore'. Yet the 'war on obesity' has hardly been won. Rates of obesity remain just as high as they were in 2007. The estimated public costs of obesity—direct to the health service and via the downstream economic effects—continue to climb, too. So how can we explain the apparent petering out of interest and attention?

In this book, I suggest that in order to understand this development, so pronounced in the case of obesity but familiar to scholars of policy more broadly, we need to take a closer look at the real 'war on obesity'—the political battle to define obesity as a public problem in need of attention across sites of democratic debate and policymaking. The key weapon in this war is knowledge, in the form first and foremost of scientific evidence. Virtually everyone engaged in the debates across Australia and Britain couches their claims in terms of 'the evidence'. From those who promote radical regulatory reform to those who deny the existence of any problem altogether, from scientific advisors to opinion columnists and patient group advocates, all actors claim to advocate for 'evidence-based' policy on obesity. There is, of course, a temptation to be cynical about this state of affairs: *they would say that, wouldn't they?* But what I want to argue here is that this universal refrain to evidence has complex, ambivalent implications, certainly more so than instinctive scepticism in policy studies and dominant accounts in (critical) public health would suggest. In important respects, the shared commitment to evidence-based policymaking (EBPM) enables democratic contestation and promotes expert and stakeholder buy-in. But I also show how the emphasis on evidence contributes to the marginalisation of obese voices, and the omission or elision of the emotive edge to this issue. And I go on to argue that this blunting of emotion should be seen in the light of the way actors also moderate and mollify their claims as they move across venues of elite and expert discussion. The result, I conclude, is a fractured, confused stalemate that risks serving the interests of the most powerful actors involved. Though these are common trends across both countries, I suggest that it is the Australian case that exhibits these pathologies more acutely and problematically—Australia's obesity debate is one that more severely excludes critical voices and that conditions actors to couch their claims in more narrowly feasible terms. This discrepancy between the cases in degree, in turn, can help to explain the factors underpinning the petering out of the 'war on obesity', and ultimately inform efforts to reignite political debate on this issue. What results is an account of obesity politics that has affinities with, and seeks to extend, some of the most exciting work on the knowledge politics of complex and contested policy issues.

To provide this more sensitive and resonant account, this book centres around two key questions: first, how do actors engaged in policy debate make sense of obesity as a problem?, and second, how and to what effect do they draw on and present these divergent interpretations across different venues of discussion? Drawing on a rich analysis of qualitative data, I identify the key narratives that actors adhere to and promote in order to make sense of this issue and underpin claims for solutions. I show how adherents to these different accounts draw on knowledge claims about the issue, revealing unique insights into how such claims conflict, cloud, and coalesce as they shift across sites of debate and over time.

I use this introductory chapter to set the scene for this analysis. I start by situating the project in the context of recent debates in policy studies about the role of expert knowledge in democratic policymaking, as well as in the context of the widening schism between mainstream and critical public health accounts of obesity politics. I do so with a view to foreshadowing the novelty of my claims, and their capacity to speak to (and challenge) these different perspectives in equal measure. I then devote a good deal of attention to outlining my approach, both because of its potential to contribute to narrative scholarship in policy studies more broadly and because of its importance in grounding the rich analysis that follows. I move on to spell out my core argument in brief, before running through the outlines of the chapters through which this argument develops. I conclude with a brief statement about what I hope and expect to achieve in making these claims.

The Politics of Policy Knowledge:
From Positions to Practices

Understanding the knowledge on which political decisions are taken has
long been perhaps *the* chief interest in policy scholarship (for the most
classic statements, see Lasswell 1951; Weiss 1977; Schon 1983; Majone
1989). Discussion in the last decade or so has centred around the notion
of 'EBPM', a legacy of the New Labour government's much-publicised
commitment to implementing 'what works'. This was a commitment
that met with sympathy and enthusiasm from some quarters in the policy
studies community (see Davies et al. 2000). But it has equally encountered fierce criticism. Some prominent scholars have lauded the prospect
of EBPM in an ideal world but remain cynical that it can amount to anything more than a fig leaf for preconceived policy in reality (see Pawson
2006). This reality, for them, is less EBPM and more 'policy-based evidence-making' (Marmot 2004). More vocal opposition still has come
from policy scholars of a more critical orientation, for whom the call for
EBPM represents a rallying cry for technocracy. Since evidence cannot be
divorced from values, they say, the effort to reduce democratic decision-
making to a dry, rational consideration of evidence must by its nature
insidiously privilege the commitments and biases of the technocratic
elite (Parsons 2002; Colebatch 2009). The controversy is largely sim-
mering now, having erupted in response to 'What works?', with EBPM
mollified to a much softer form of 'evidence-informed' policymaking for
even its keenest proponents (e.g. Head 2010). But the debate should not
be understood as settled. In fact, it represents a continuation of a long-
standing dispute about the right place of expert knowledge in the policy
process. This debate over whose knowledge ought to count, and over how
and where such knowledge ought to be represented, is one with positions
long staked out.

Yet in more recent years dedicated work on the politics of policy knowledge has, if not breached this impasse, skirted around it. This is work that
is less concerned with ideological statements about the role of evidence
in policymaking, and more grounded in rich and detailed study of policy
practices and the manner in which they incorporate relevant forms of

knowledge. This is not to say it is objective or value free—indeed, such work is for the most part interpretive or critical in nature, and thereby rejects or repudiates the very notion of objectivity (for this tradition, see especially Fischer and Forester 1993; Fischer 2000, 2003, 2009; Fischer and Gottweis 2012). But in its focus on practices, rather than polemicising, it opens up greater space for mutual engagement and interpretation about the politics of policy knowledge. This work often engages in the concepts and tools of science and technology studies (see Hoppe 1999, 2010), and its scholars therefore appreciate the nuanced, variegated relationship between the scientific and other sources and forms of knowledge and power in political affairs (e.g. Lahsen 2008; Dunlop 2014; Wesselink and Hoppe 2011). It moves past the reductive dichotomy between democracy and technocracy to examine the interaction between different sorts of experts and elites and the complex configurations of power through which technical expertise manifests, conflicts, and coalesces (e.g. Freeman and Sturdy 2014; Strassheim and Kettunen 2014). It goes 'beyond EBPM' to reveal the complex ways in which expert knowledge interacts with, and becomes mediated by, other claims to legitimate influence in policy work (e.g. Fischer 1995; Smith 2013). It is this exciting and growing branch of scholarship that I seek to build on in this book.

The politics of obesity represents an excellent case through which to make such a contribution, especially in relation to the two countries in my analysis. It is the rapid rise (and relative plateau or fall) of obesity on the agenda in Australia and the UK, and the hotly contested knowledge politics surrounding the issue in both countries underpinning these dynamics, that makes these contexts so interesting. Defined officially as a body mass index (BMI) of 30 or higher,[1] obesity has emerged as an important issue in public health policymaking in these countries as elsewhere over the last three decades (see Wang et al. 2011; WHO 2000). But with this rise, there has been little prospect of consensus among experts, politicians, lobbyists, and non-governmental organisations (NGOs), among others,

---

[1] BMI is a measurement (mass in kilograms divided by height in metres squared) by which individuals can be classified, with a calculation over 30 considered obese, and over 25 deemed overweight. It was initially applied by epidemiologists to understand public health trends but has become a common tool in medical practice as well. There is much controversy surrounding the crudeness of the measure and its applicability to different individuals and populations.

about its nature, its causes, and the appropriate public policy response. Obesity is, firstly, an issue of considerable contestation, on both ideological and material grounds (Dixon and Broom 2007). There are clashing philosophies about the role of the state; there are also a multitude of interests involved, including the powerful food and pharmaceutical industries, competing expert and professional groups, patient activists, and so on. Obesity is, secondly, an issue of great scientific uncertainty. Little is known about the relationship of obesity to health outcomes and even less known about the capacity of government to intervene (Botterill and Hindmoor 2012). And, finally, obesity is an issue of immense complexity (Foresight 2007). It cuts across a range of different specialties and disciplines, both within health and beyond (see Kelly 2009). And in policy terms it inevitably involves an array of interrelated causal factors that can be hard to disentangle and make sense of (Lang and Rayner 2007).

Yet in spite of this conflict, uncertainty, and complexity, 'the evidence' remains absolutely central to debate both in Australia and in the UK. These obesity debates therefore represent what Bent Flyvbjerg (2006), in his passionate defence of case study research, calls 'extreme cases'. The very centrality of 'the evidence' to such contested, uncertain, and complex policy terrains makes them fascinating exemplars through which to understand knowledge politics. They can throw into sharp relief ongoing questions and dilemmas in the relevant literature about how actors draw on knowledge to make sense of issues and advance their claims in political debate.

Furthermore, the comparison between the cases becomes valuable in drawing such inferences, albeit not necessarily in the way I expected or that typifies comparative case study work. [2] In practice, I found rather more similarities than differences across the cases, and much of what I have to say applies equally to both debates. Yet precisely because the countries share broadly similar epistemic and political cultures, and because the content of the debate bears so many similarities, the few discrepancies I note, largely around the more effective institutional channelling of

---

[2] This is entirely in keeping with the norms of interpretive research, where preconceived concepts or categories can melt away, to be replaced by new ideas and themes that emerge inductively during fieldwork (see Hendriks 2007; Flyvbjerg 2006).

debate and thus promotion of ongoing contestation and scrutiny in the British case, are especially important. This allows fruitful discussion in the concluding chapters about policy processes and their links to knowledge and representation.

But before getting too far ahead with these intricacies, it is important to acknowledge that much academic interest has already been shown in the politics of obesity in recent years, both in the two countries I look at and beyond. However, the story I uncover here, and the dynamics underpinning it, remains very much understudied and unappreciated. As it stands, scholars from within and outside public health recite incompatible accounts of obesity politics. For the former, the key message—one linked to policy studies cynicism about the obstruction and obfuscation of EBPM—is that 'politicisation' has got in the way of dealing with obesity: that it is an issue beyond the governing capabilities of political actors addicted to short-term, siloed thinking, beholden to the powerful food lobby and cowed by the prospect of perceived Nanny State-ism (see Brownell and Battle Horgen 2003; Swinburn et al. 2011; Lang and Rayner 2012; Egger and Swinburn 2012). For the latter, the key message—one that resonates more with critical opposition to the very goal of EBPM in policy scholarship—is that obesity has been subject to sustained efforts towards 'depoliticisation': that the zealous—even 'micro-fascist' (see Rail et al. 2010)—public health lobby have sought to impose anti-obesity measures in the absence of compelling evidence and appropriate public consultation (Campos 2004; Oliver 2005; Gard and Wright 2001; Botterill and Hindmoor 2012; Saguy 2013). There is insight of value in both accounts. However, both remain caricatured representations of the knowledge politics of this issue. Both are insufficiently attentive to the complex interactions between actors across different sites of debate—the range of knowledge claims brought to bear on the issue in different contexts by different actors. Both, in their determination to, respectively, build up and knock down obesity as a policy issue, have overlooked the ebbing of attention and impetus for policy action and the reasons underlying the rise and (relative) fall of obesity on the public agenda.

As such, the story recounted in this book provides a vital corrective to these categorical accounts. But it also goes beyond these (mainly) narrow accounts of obesity as an exceptional or important issue in its own right and situates debate about this issue more clearly in the field of policy studies alongside other similarly complex and contested fields. The more nuanced account offered here has strong affinities with important contemporary work on 'wicked' problems (see Rittel and Webber 1973; APSC 2007), in particular on how actors draw on and beyond scientific evidence to advocate for policy solutions in the face of uncertainty and complexity (see, e.g. Lahsen 2008; Monaghan 2011; Smith 2013; Griggs and Howarth 2013). Over the course of the chapters that follow, it draws on the knowledge politics of obesity to contribute to long-standing concerns in policy and politics scholarship about agenda-setting, issue management, conflict neutralisation, democratic representation, and policy implementation, among others. And as such, though it presents a richly grounded thick description of the obesity debates in Britain and Australia, its insights also speak to a much broader audience beyond those concerned with public health.

Orientation and Approach

If the watchword of this book is nuance—set up as my account is against the polemical or cynical opposition to EBPM generally, and between the radical 'politicised' and 'depoliticised' accounts of obesity's knowledge politics specifically—then this almost certainly relates to my entry to the field. The 'politicised' camp tends to be composed of public health experts, with a strong normative commitment to winning the substantive 'war on obesity' and neutering the perceived power of the biggest obstacle, the wealthy food lobby. The 'depoliticised' camp, in contrast, is informed by a feminist or sociological critique incensed by the 'war on obesity's' perceived reproduction of 'fat hatred' or 'victim blaming'. Both represent overtly political interventions, designed to promote a particular set of policy outcomes, and indeed both closely approximate to important narratives in the public debate on this issue that I uncover in my analysis.

My project, in contrast, began as a theoretical enterprise—an interest in how narrative manifests in, and affects the prospects of, deliberative governance (see Boswell 2013 for a lengthy exposition)—and obesity emerged as the case through which to explore it. I struck upon it, for the reasons outlined above, because it appealed as such an interesting case through which to explore my theoretical ruminations. Britain and Australia appealed as a useful comparison to add layers of nuance to my analysis. Interesting and useful such choices have proven, though not entirely for the reasons I initially thought, as alluded to above. In any case, I was, in the initial stages, agnostic about obesity itself and I remain somewhat ambivalent about the competing interpretations of the issue that I present in this book. Of course, I do not find all the narratives equally compelling—the reactionary Nanny State account in particular I find quite discomforting—but I remain attracted to aspects of all the other accounts. And in the process of unpacking these interpretations, I have also developed a strong empathy for the chief concerns or motivators of *both* politicised and depoliticised scholarly accounts of obesity politics. Yet I remain convinced that neither adequately captures the uncertainty and complexity that pervade this debate, and so I have set about trying to rectify these oversights in this book.

Meanwhile, much of the terminology of deliberative governance that inspired my initial inquiry has been stripped away in this rendering of my analysis. The rationale is that doing so can ease the clutter of concepts and engage more forthrightly with relevant debates in policy studies and public health. However, readers should be aware that its ghost very much continues to haunt my account (see Boswell forthcoming especially for this angle). My orientation, in line with the commitments associated with deliberative governance, is to process rather than outcome. My concern is neither to solve obesity nor to dispel it as a concept or category, but to ensure that the political debate on the issue remains vibrant, fair, and inclusive.

The tools by which I went about this task were drawn from the tradition of interpretive policy studies. As an analyst I am, in this sense, primarily interested in the ways in which the actors involved make sense of this complex problem and recount their experiences in working to influence policy work that addresses it (see the contributions of Yanow and Schwartz-Shea 2006; Bevir and Rhodes 2010; Yanow and Schwartz-Shea 2012). The key tool I take from this box is narrative policy analysis, an approach which seeks to identify and reconstruct the narratives that actors rely on to make sense of and argue about complex and contested issues (see Roe 1994; Stone 2002; Fischer 2003; Boswell 2013). Most of the empirical work adopting this notion in politics and policy studies has been either on uncovering the content of narratives on specific policy controversies (e.g. Boswell et al. 2011) or on identifying how political actors construct narratives to gain consent or assure legitimacy for their actions (e.g. Grube 2012; Dye 2014). The former approach largely divests actors of their agency. The latter risks seeing them as masterly over the rhetoric they produce. Both potentially render narrative as something that can be ascertained as a singular text. I therefore favour a middle ground which recognises that political actors operate in the context of pre-existing narratives, but equally that they have capacity to reinterpret and reconfigure these narratives in context (Boswell 2013). Narratives exist, but not independent of agents (Stone 2002; Bevir and Rhodes 2003). They must be brought to life in and for a specific context, reproduced and rearticulated by embedded political actors. They require narration.

Seeking to understand narration meant grappling with the recent turn to dramaturgy and performance in policy studies. My work here builds especially on recent scholarship that draws on these insights about dramaturgy and performance to shed new light on the knowledge politics of democratic contestation over health policymaking (see Greenhalgh and Russell 2006; Boswell et al. 2015). This is a turn that has been pioneered in the recent work of Maarten Hajer (2005, 2009), though it also has clear affinities with recent interpretive work in rhetoric (see Gottweis 2007; Finlayson 2007) and draws heavily on the seminal works of scholars such as Burke (1969), Goffman (1959), and Edelman (1964) who underpin this tradition. Hajer's concern is in going beyond mere discursive artefacts to understand better how the material and relational contexts of interactions in policy debate condition and affect the discursive. As such, in order to understand the dramaturgical context of narration, I had to establish where key policy debate on obesity happened and how it unfolded.

This involved in the first place a process of mapping the obesity debates in both countries. I worked with key informants in initial 'helicopter interviews' (Hajer 2006)—informal interviews prior to beginning my formal fieldwork, speaking with actors well established in the area who could, as the name suggests, provide a broad oversight on the policy issue and its dimensions. Based on these interviews and extensive background reading, I set about identifying the crucial sites of debate across both cases. These were venues that involved a mix of different actors, invoked different sorts of norms, and had different (but also, in their own way, important) roles in informing policy work on this issue. The sites listed below occupied my focus over the timeframe from 2007, when the issue peaked on the public agenda, to 2013, when I finished conducting fieldwork. Table 1.1 provides a brief summary and rundown of the data acquired in each context, but I flesh them out in some detail below to give greater richness to the analysis that follows.

Table 1.1 Mapping the obesity debates in Britain and Australia

	Australia	Britain
Data gathered and analysed	Approx. 1100 documents, 11 hours of video footage, and 25 interviews with policy actors	Approx. 500 documents, 12 hours of video footage, and 11 interviews with policy actors
Mass media Articles, opinion pieces, and letters to the editor on obesity (2007–2012)	Approx. 500 articles from across the *Age*, the *Sydney Morning Herald*, the *Australian*, the *Daily Telegraph*, and the *Sun-Herald*, interviews with 1 journalist and 14 public advocates	Approx. 250 articles from across the *Guardian*, the *Telegraph*, the *Daily Mail*, the *Sun*, interviews with 7 public advocates
Taskforce Expert report commissioned by government on costs of and solutions to the obesity crisis	*National Preventative Health Taskforce (2008/2009)* Reports and government response, submissions, consultation notes, interviews with 3 Taskforce members	*Foresight (2007)* Report and related documentation, interviews with 2 participants, interview with 1 member of expert advisory committee
Collaborative network Involving government officials, food industry representatives, and public health advocates	*Food and Health Dialogue* Communiqués, website, interviews with 3 Dialogue members	*Public Health Responsibility Deals* Website, interview with 1 Responsibility Deal member

(continued)

Table 1.1 (continued)

	Australia	Britain
Democratic innovations New institutional arrangements designed to foster public deliberation (with obesity one issue among many up for discussion)	*2020 Summit* Australia's 'best and brightest' discuss critical issues facing the nation, including a stream on health (of just under 100 members): – Report and government response, session notes and 3 hours' of video footage, interviews with 2 participants	*Food Standards Agency's Open Board Meetings* The community board holds 10 'open' meetings every year broadcast live on television and archived on the Internet: – Video footage, meeting agendas, and minutes
Parliamentary inquiries	– House of Representatives' Inquiry into Obesity (2008/2009): report and response, submissions, Hansard, and interviews with 2 MPs and 7 witnesses – Senate Inquiry into Protecting Children from Junk Food Advertising (2009): reports, submissions, Hansard, video footage, and interviews with 1 senator and 2 witnesses	

The Australian Debate

The Mass Media

This site was universally acknowledged as crucial by the actors themselves engaged in this debate, but it is of course in itself much too broad and unruly to examine in its entirety. Faced with this complexity, I opted to analyse newspaper coverage as something of a proxy for the broader public sphere. I analysed a range of tabloid and broadsheet, and progressive and conservative newspapers, coding over 500 articles from across relatively progressive metropolitan broadsheets like the *Age* and the *Sydney Morning Herald*, the more conservative national broadsheet the *Australian*, and conservative metropolitan tabloids the *Sun-Herald* and the *Daily Telegraph*.

The 2020 Summit

This was an initiative of the then newly elected Rudd Labor government. It involved a meeting of the nation's 'best and brightest' minds early in April 2008 to discuss the major issues facing Australia. One stream was specifically set aside for health issues, and obesity was a major theme of these deliberations. The physical setting was an opening of the doors to Parliament—one thought to distinguish the new Labor government from its notoriously closed-off predecessor (Davis 2008). After a call for nominations, the government invited 1000 experts and celebrities to participate in intensive group interactions, 86 of them in the Health Stream. Innovation was welcomed and participants were encouraged to challenge the status quo.

The National Preventative Health Taskforce

Headed by a committee of nine well-known public and primary health experts, it was established by the Minister to recommend 'evidence-based strategies' for improving preventative health around smoking, alcohol abuse, and obesity. The Taskforce held committee meetings, sub-committee meetings, technical group meetings, and regional consultations. It was an expert-dominated site, with only researcher and practitioner input sought in intensive deliberations (HoR Inquiry, February 4 2009, p. 8). Other interested parties could send written submissions to the Taskforce, of which they received over 400. An advisory report

(Preventative Health Taskforce 2009) and technical paper (Preventative Health Taskforce 2008) were the key outputs.

The House of Representatives' (HoR) Weighing It up Inquiry into Obesity

The terms of reference for this inquiry were put by the Minister before the Standing Committee on Health and Ageing in early 2008. It received hundreds of written submissions. The main focus of my analysis was on the 16 public hearings held in a dozen locations, including major cities and some regional centres. These hearings, fully transcribed in Hansard, pitted the Committee members in intimate conversation with stakeholders and experts. Proceedings were open to interested members of the public.

The Inquiry into Banning Junk Food Advertising to Children

This inquiry resulted from a Private Member's Bill launched by Senator Bob Brown, then leader of the Australian Greens Party. The inquiry received fewer than two dozen submissions and had just one public hearing at Parliament. This inquiry produced two reports—a majority one against the Bill and a minority one for it.

The Food and Health Dialogue

This is a government-led body that incorporates industry and public health representatives. It emerged in 2009. The setting is a committee room in Parliament. The interactive, intensive deliberations within this site have occurred very much behind closed doors, with low-profile communiqués the only form of publicity. Participants are cast as problem-solvers, tasked with being pragmatic and collaborative in their outlook.

The British Debate

The Mass Media

As in Australia, the public sphere in the UK is a noisy, messy series of over-lapping sites. In fact, in the UK it is considerably noisier and messier—with a much bigger and more diverse news media, as well as a more active civil society and a larger informal public sphere through social media and interpersonal networking. To get an appropriate sense of the breadth of narratives expressed in this arena, I narrowed my focus down to key newspaper publications in an attempt to echo what I had done in Australia. Adopting the same approach, I identified and examined 250 articles from across the *Guardian*, a progressive broadsheet, the *Telegraph*, a conservative broadsheet, the *Daily Mail*, a conservative tabloid, and the left-wing tabloid the *Mirror*.

The Foresight Process

The Foresight report was produced by a select group of public health and other technical experts after a lengthy process of research and discussion. Like the Taskforce in Australia, it was a process dominated by experts in that its steering committee only sought to consult with renowned public health academics and practitioners. They were tasked with modelling the future prevalence and costs of obesity, breaking down and explaining the causes of the problem, and pointing the way towards potential solutions. Soon after the report was published, an expert advisory committee was set up, featuring many of the experts who had played a role in crafting the report.

The Board Meetings of the Food Standards Agency (FSA)

The FSA had been set up as a body at arm's-length from the Department of Health in the aftermath of the bovine spongiform encephalopathy (BSE or 'mad cow disease') scandal in the 1990s. So, though not set up specifically to deliberate on obesity, the issue quickly became one of the key items in the board's remit. It has been an important site of political discussion and policy work on obesity, in particular making high-profile and at times controversial pushes for traffic light labelling and firmer food reformulation targets. The board features a diverse range of experts and community representatives, a move the government is seen to have made especially to ward off suspicions of cronyism which had dogged the making and implementation of food policy previously. More unusually, given this history, it was decided that board meetings should be open to the public. The board therefore gets together every month on an ongoing basis to deliberate on food-related issues in front of a live audience. The event is broadcast and archived over the Internet for anyone to view.

The Public Health Responsibility Deals

Established by the coalition government in 2010, the Deals were set up to take over many of the points removed from the responsibility of the FSA in the belief that the agency had become too political (Lang 2010). The stated purpose of the Deals has been to promote cooperation among industry, government, NGOs, and experts on persistent social problems around alcohol and tobacco control and, of greatest interest to me, physical activity and nutrition. These ongoing arrangements bring together participants in strategic meetings on a monthly or bi-monthly basis. Participants are cast as problem-solvers and are expected to be constructive and pragmatic in their discussions. Discussions occur strictly behind closed doors, with the intention of giving participants space to discuss the issues free from the glare of publicity.

Outline of the Argument

Ultimately, based on lengthy immersion in the vast wealth of data stemming from these sites, I developed an analysis of six competing policy narratives that order debate on this issue across both cases (though only five are salient in Australia), and assessed how and to what effect these narratives move across these diverse policy settings. The focus was not, as I have explained, on reconstructing these policy narratives as dead, fixed 'texts', but in bringing them to life by establishing how the actors engaged in debate and policy work perform the narratives that they subscribe to in and across particular venues (see Boswell 2016, ahead-of-print). Such an analysis, I hope to show, is attentive to the way that policy actors define the parameters of the issue and characterise the groups and interests involved, draw together scientific evidence with other sources of knowledge on obesity, and inflame, reconcile, or at times obscure areas of ethical and interest-based conflict in policymaking.

This analysis produces a novel, nuanced account of obesity politics which sits in between the black-and-white 'politicised' and 'depoliticised' interpretations which dominate the current understanding of the construction of obesity as a political issue. Along the way, it debunks or complicates other common presumptions within social scientific scholarship on public health. It reveals that the parsimonious framing of debate in behavioural versus environmental terms remains inattentive to the nuanced overlap and intersection of behavioural and environmental—not to mention biomedical, socio-economic, and cultural—factors in the accounts that political actors adhere to and advocate. It shows that the debate is not just about competing interpretations of what to do about the problem, but about the scope of the problem or the fact that there is even a problem at all.

More important still, this is an analysis that extends and, at times, challenges emerging work on similarly complex or wicked issues and the influence of science and expertise on policy work in these areas. These findings will be of interest to those working in, and at times draw on concepts from, science and technology studies. But the key contributions are to ongoing discussions and debates within the literature on policymaking and democratic governance, particularly as this work pertains to the place, use, and interpretation of policy-relevant knowledge. So, I contribute to burgeoning literature on the subtleties of democratic representation in a context of networked governance, showing that the representation of knowledge can be as significant as the knowledge claims themselves. I provide nuanced insights into the persistent appeal of EBPM, challenging orthodox claims that such a goal need be associated with the exclusion of democratic contestation or the corruption or crass manipulation of science, while outlining more subtle, but equally pervasive and problematic consequences of a 'fetish' for evidence. And I provide fresh insights into the political dynamics of issue containment, showing how knowledge claims become fractured and nebulous as actors move across sites of debate towards elite and empowered institutions of policymaking.

The overarching story that emerges is of political contests mired by stalemate over the 'evidence' in both cases, though to varying degrees. Academic, professional, and activist proponents of all the competing narratives feel compelled to couch their claims primarily in scientific terms—a state of affairs that ensures mutual engagement and reciprocity, but which crowds out the voice of the affected public at the very centre of this issue, obese people themselves, elides or marginalises the emotional edge to this issue, and generates a haze of contested and confusing knowledge claims on the issue. I show how the powerful food lobby can capitalise on, but not entirely create or control, the resultant ambiguity. In the meantime, there is a noticeable blunting of the force of critical or urgent voices, masking of key aspects of conflict on this issue, and undercutting of claims for significant policy change, all away from effective scrutiny. The policy outcome is a worst-of-all-worlds compromise. The focus is on highly visible policies (such as social marketing) that disappoint the public health lobby while still perpetuating the responsibilisation and 'victim-blaming' which so concern more critical actors. Of even greater concern is the political outcome—a sense of a stalled debate which leaves many of its participants despondent about the future. The risk is that with the policy 'war on obesity' all but over, the political 'war' rumbles on only intermittently, further in the background, and with little apparent hope of resolution. This risk, I find, is more acutely realised in the Australian case, where critical voices are blatantly excluded from elite debate and actors themselves reflect openly on conditioning and mollifying their claims for fear of not being taken seriously. I conclude by arguing that the differences between these cases, focusing especially on the practices in the British case that somewhat better enable ongoing political contestation and scrutiny, provide some basis on which to envision governing institutions and practices for a brighter future. This is not, to be clear, a future where the fabled 'war on obesity' in substantive terms is likely to succeed in Britain and Australia, but a future where the real 'war on obesity'—the political contest over the nature and meaning of this issue—might be allowed to carry on in more inclusive terms, and on a more even footing.

Structure of the Book

What follows below is a breakdown of how I construct this argument over the course of the book. It is, in broad terms, divided into two parts, with each devoted to answering the broad anchoring research questions outlined at the outset of this chapter. I outline both below.

Part 1: Problem Definition

Part 1 focuses on how actors make sense of obesity as a policy problem. Here I identify and outline the competing policy narratives on this issue, working to draw out the key discrepancies and disagreements among them. The result is an analysis that challenges prevailing assumptions and existing academic wisdom about the social construction of obesity as a policy problem. Just as importantly, it sheds new light on topics of interest in policy and politics scholarship, augmenting the literature on discursive politics and linking it to perennial concerns in this field about the battle over issue scope and the competition to set and control the public agenda.

Chapter 2 focuses on the pair of narratives which constitute the primary public debate in both countries, in that they are the most prominent accounts with the largest backing. The key point is that both centre around the question of individual agency, though not in the way that much of the existing literature on the social construction of obesity (and similar issues) typically suggests. The contest to understand the issue of obesity here is not, as usually represented in this literature, a simple one of 'structure versus agency' or 'environment versus behaviour'; instead, it is a more complex contest between narratives which mobilise features across the broader discourses associated with the 'environmental' and the 'behavioural'. I find that as actors perform the key competing narratives on obesity, they place different levels of emphasis on these factors in explaining and working to solve the problem. The dominant narrative underpinning policy in both countries—Facilitated Agency—sees obesity as a problem caused largely by broad environmental factors, but promotes the most elegant and feasible solution as working to better enable individuals to manage their own weight. Proponents of this account thus advocate providing some appropriate support from government and other societal actors, but overall they place primary emphasis on the need for policy to promote behaviour change at an individual level. Structured Opportunity, the primary counternarrative, voiced by public health experts and activists, accepts that behavioural explanations of the obesity epidemic must be 'part of the mix', but it nevertheless sees the major policy gains to be had at a population level in regulating the food environment. Both, ultimately, claim to advocate making 'healthy choices easier' in the contest for the middle ground; the broader lesson being that performing political narratives in practice represents less a perfect or pure manifestation of a distinct discourse, and more an effort to 'bridge' distinct discourses in order to better mobilise broader support.

Chapter 3 further drills down to distil the divergent accounts of obesity promoted by scientists and medical professionals: the Individual Intervention and Social Dislocation narratives. These are narratives that are more specialised or niche, and which are marginal in the broader media debate, but which are becoming increasingly prevalent in more elite or expert-dominated policy settings—albeit, and instructive of the arguments to follow later in the book, that the latter remains only latent in the Australian context, adhered to privately by key experts but never emphasised publicly in consequential venues of policy discussion. Both narratives seek to reimagine the scope of this issue. The Individual Intervention narrative stresses a focus on treating individuals who are already obese. The essence of this account, then, entails a narrowed focus on the 'downstream' consequences of obesity for individual health. In contrast, for adherents to the Social Dislocation narrative, the focus should extend beyond the typical 'environmental' focus on food markets and opportunities for exercise to the wider social and economic determinants of ill-health. Obesity, for them, is just one particularly visible and visceral manifestation of modern society's inequalities and dysfunctions, and therefore nothing much can really be done to halt its spread. As such, this chapter challenges, indeed inverts, the orthodox assumption in policy studies that those seeking to expand the scope of a policy issue demand tangible change, and that those seeking to narrow it merely reinforce the status quo. In the broader context of the book's argument, though, the key contribution here is to draw out the ways in which these accounts diverge from or extend the mainstream debate articulated in Chap. 2. I begin the task of highlighting the epistemic rivalries that exist between competing specialists in this area, and the effects that such rivalries, and the uncertainties they engender, have on expert advocacy.

Chapter 4 looks beyond the mainstream and established experts to constructions of obesity at the margins, which dispute the nature or very existence of this purported problem. These are narratives that, contra the usual focus on the efforts of civil society actors to gain attention for their issue, actively seek to push obesity *off* the public agenda. Intriguingly, my analysis here identifies two narratives that push in this direction, only from opposite ends of the spectrum. One is a Nanny State account, associated with a reactionary worldview, that cautions against state involvement of any kind and which, contra prevailing wisdom, is almost (in the British case) or completely (in the Australian case) confined to the fringes of the press. The other marginal account, in contrast, is a Moral Panic narrative founded in activist critique and critical social science of public health. The Moral Panic narrative questions the extent or even existence of the obesity epidemic. I show that though this is a prevalent narrative among social activists, it is one that, like the Nanny State account, is seen to lack credibility within established expert committees and other policymaking venues. The analysis in this sense brings to light processes of exclusion and marginalisation in the contest over the public agenda that can limit the range of 'credible' narratives expressed in elite or formal policy settings, especially in the Australian case where proponents of the Moral Panic narrative have been actively shut out from sites of elite policy discussion.

Part 2: Policy Engagement

With Part 1 having set out the nature of the debate and the competing interpretations that prevail within it, Part 2 looks at the implications for policy work on obesity. It focuses on how proponents of the competing policy narratives on obesity perform their preferred account across sites of policy debate and expert and stakeholder engagement. The themes that emerge centre around the place, use, and interpretation of the key weapon in the political 'war on obesity'—expert knowledge. Each chapter looks, respectively, at how knowledge is represented, claimed, contested, and transmitted in these debates.

Chapter 5 is inspired by the most lasting impression from my analysis of the data; my observation that almost all of the proponents of the narratives recounted in Part 1—at least as expressed in formal or elite sites of debate—are themselves lean and fit. As such, here I look at how and to what effect the proponents of the competing narratives, usually experts of one sort or another, claim to speak on behalf of the most affected public in this instance, obese people themselves. I identify three key sets of representative claims—as Carer, Nanny, and Role Model—mobilised as actors perform their preferred narrative across both countries. The first is based on an emotional attachment built up through a close relationship between professional experts and the obese individuals in their care. The second is, in contrast, built around the absence of any close connection, and instead based on a stern and detached assessment of what is in obese people's best interests. The third is grounded in experience—expert advocates serve to publicise and even themselves model 'healthy' behaviour which (as they perceive it) confused or put-upon obese people might not fully understand otherwise. Though each claim expresses a large degree of empathy for the obese, my analysis suggests that they work collectively in both cases to undermine these good intentions by denying obese individuals' agency and by blunting the emotional edge to this issue. The findings in this chapter therefore link to an emerging body of scholarship which emphasises the role of ordinary citizens, and affect and emotion, in democratic representation and policy work.

Chapter 6 is inspired by the biggest initial impression from my field-work—the tendency of all actors in both countries, regardless of the narrative they adhere to, to place central emphasis on the value of scientific evidence and the hopes of EBPM in regard to this issue. I drill down in this chapter into how these actors claim knowledge. What I reveal challenges prevailing assumptions, prominent especially among critical policy scholars in general (and equally prominent among critical scholars of obesity in particular), that such an orientation serves to 'depoliticise' this issue and render it a matter for technocratic problem-solving. In contrast, I highlight that the apparent 'fetish' for evidence does not negate other sources of knowledge, and that actors actually weave together all sorts of 'policy-relevant knowledge' (Tenbensel 2006), including normative claims, cultural wisdom, and practical (especially professional) experience. I also show that these actors are highly reflexive about their use of science and about the limits to EBPM. Yet I maintain that the emphasis on evidence retains an important but largely unheralded downside—chiefly that it subordinates the lived experience of this issue in both countries, and mutes or numbs the emotional side of this issue. This, I foreshadow, is especially important in the context of the stalemate over the evidence and the tendency of advocates to mute and moderate knowledge claims as they approach empowered sites of decision-making, covered in the two chapters to come.

Chapter 7 builds on this work by focusing on how actors contest knowledge claims about obesity. I show how the conflicting narratives on obesity typically order actors' accounts of what facts matter, how they should be interpreted, and how they ought to inform policymaking. But what I also show is that these narratives can equally be seen as *conflicted* to some degree along these dimensions. Actors do no neatly subscribe to a narrative and arrange their evidence in service of a cleaner and more coherent account—there is no simplistic vision of mere 'policy-based evidence-making' in which actors deliberately or rationally assemble convenient facts to buttress their position. My more fine-grained analysis reveals inconsistencies and incompatibilities across these collective accounts. Indeed, I uncover a haze of overlapping knowledge claims which can be incoherent and confusing, not least for the actors involved themselves. I argue that the result in both countries, ultimately, is broad agreement on what ought to count as knowledge on obesity in general but disagreement and confusion about what that knowledge specifically means for policymaking on this issue. These findings contribute significantly to contemporary debates about 'EBPM' in the policy studies literature, offering a much more nuanced account of what a commitment to EBPM looks like in practice and novel insights into both positive and negative democratic implications.

Chapter 8 assesses the ways in which experts and advocates promote their preferred narratives across sites of policy work and debate, most especially as they become engaged in elite settings associated with formal decision-making. I show in this chapter how the norms embedded in such formal institutions shape these actors' claims to, and claims on the basis of, expert knowledge. The point is that policy narratives are not voiced in a contextual vacuum—they must contend with the 'sacred stories' of established political institutions and policy practices. My account in particular showcases the ways in which these intersubjectively understood contextual factors impact on the performance of narratives in subtly different ways across the cases. What I find in broad terms is that the manner in which actors give voice to their preferred narrative invariably softens and loses specificity over time and across these diffuse sites of engagement. In line with the findings in Chaps. 4 and 5, I show that this is especially pronounced in the Australian case, where advocates are more likely to condition their claims in line with what they perceive to be 'feasible' in elite and empowered settings, and then have almost no opportunity to revisit or scrutinise policy work 'downstream'. The result is that any calls for significant policy reform become watered down, providing 'wriggle room' that powerful actors can exploit in the absence of high-profile scrutiny, conflict, and contestation. The findings therefore make important contributions to long-standing debates about conflict and ambiguity in policy work.

In the Conclusion, I show that what emerges from the analysis is the picture of a stalled 'war on obesity'. I show that the continued deference to scientific evidence, and the impact that this has on the way expert advocates interact with each other, the public, and the policymakers they are trying to convince, results in a confusing stalemate, with little by way of tangible policy action or continued public concern. It not only engenders an inadequate policy response, it also removes the impetus for further contestation and debate. As such, this conclusion focuses on the lessons that can be gleaned from this analysis in order to reignite policy debate and ensure greater attention and scrutiny for this issue. I stress four lessons in particular, which can be more neatly conceptualised in two pairs. The first pair involve bringing the emotive side of this issue to the fore throughout the debate, having shown through my analysis that it remains hidden or sidelined in both cases. As such, I advocate moving beyond expert delegates, and instead promote the value in *affective embodiment*, via efforts to ensure that obese individuals have a visible presence and audible voice across sites of debate. I also advocate a concerted effort to produce and disseminate more social science evidence on the *emotions* of obese individuals, with a view that doing so will sustain visceral, affective discussion of the lived experience of obesity in expert and elite settings of policy debate. The second pair involve better sustaining democratic contestation through the policy process. They are based in particular on key discrepancies between the two cases, with the problems I identify being more acute or widespread in the Australian context than the British one. First, I emphasise the importance of structuring and practising policy debate in a way that emphasises the contingency and ambiguity of policy compromise, and affords opponents in civil society ample opportunity and impetus to voice ongoing reservations or grievances. Second, and related, I emphasise the importance of helping such actors to effectively 'stay' with the issue through the policy process, so that they can better scrutinise the way ambiguous, contingent compromise is actually put into action.

A Word on 'Impact'

The argument as I build it through the book is complex and multifaceted. It confronts along the way a number of important assumptions in the policy studies and (critical) public health literatures, wrestling with prevailing ideas about the social construction of problems, policy advocacy, issue containment, EBPM, affective politics, democratic representation, stigma, and beyond. This is a book that began, as I explain above, as a highly esoteric exercise in operationalising strictly theoretical concerns, and, despite its subsequent iterations of evolution, it surely remains richly conceptual as an enterprise.

However, I want to stress before getting into the analysis that my concerns here are not, if they ever really were, strictly academic. It is not possible to engage in such detail with an issue—with the richly detailed narratives about it and with the people who passionately perform those narratives in public debate—without making some sort of personal investment. And so I hope that this book, and particularly the key findings and suggestions outlined in its Conclusion, will generate genuine 'impact' on the knowledge politics of obesity in Australia and the UK, as with elsewhere and perhaps more broadly in relation to similarly complex and contested issues. To be clear, the expectation is not that even adopting wholesale the key reforms that my accounts build to will win the 'war on obesity' for policy analysts. Indeed, if anything my stance remains that nothing can possibly solve obesity. That is precisely the point about 'wicked' policy problems. Indeed, perhaps as might apply uniquely among such policy problems, I remain ambivalent about whether solving obesity is even a desirable goal. Nor, for that matter, is my expectation that even taking full heed of my suggestions will enable the public health lobby to win the political 'war on obesity'. There remain obvious, well-documented political obstacles to that eventuality, as there are with respect to many of the most complex and contested problems that policymakers deal with.

What I hope my account will contribute, however, is to help raise the profile of obesity as an issue of government attention again. This hope is not, to be clear, for any particular set of regulations to prevail, but simply for the current, worst-of-all-words stalemate to be reinterrogated and shaken up. The take-home message of the book is that though the policy 'war on obesity' may never be won, it is possible for the political war to be fought in a more sustained fashion on a more even footing. For that impact to occur, though, it is essential to first establish a better understanding of the dynamics of that war. And it is to this that my attention turns first, in Part 1 of the book.

References

Australian Public Service Commission (APSC). (2007). *Tackling wicked problems: A public policy perspective*. Canberra: Australian Government, APSC.

Bevir, M., & Rhodes, R. A. W. (2003). *Interpreting British governance*. London: Routledge.

Bevir, M., & Rhodes, R. A. W. (2010). *The state as cultural practice*. Oxford: Oxford University Press.

Boswell, C., Geddes, A., & Scholten, P. (2011). The role of narratives in migration policy-making: A research framework. *British Journal of Politics and International Relations, 13*(1), 1–11.

Boswell, J. (2013). Why and how narrative matters in deliberative systems. *Political Studies, 61*(3), 620–636.

Boswell, J. (2016, Ahead-of-Print). "The performance of political narratives: How Britain and Australia's 'fat bombs' fizzled out." *British Journal of Politics and International Relations*. DOI: 10.1177/1369148116630232.

Boswell, J. (forthcoming). Deliberating downstream: Countering democratic distortions in the policy process. *Perspectives on Politics*.

Boswell, J., Settle, C., & Dugdale, A. (2015). Who speaks, and in what voice? The challenge of engaging the 'public' in health policy decision-making. *Public Management Review, 17*(9), 1358–1374.

Botterill, L., & Hindmoor, A. (2012). Turtles all the way down: Bounded rationality in an evidence-based age. *Policy Studies, 33*(5), 367–379.

Brownell, K. D., & Battle Horgen, K. (2003). *Food fight: The inside story of the food industry, America's obesity crisis and what we can do about it*. New York: McGraw-Hill.

Burke, K (1969). *A rhetoric of motives*. University of California Press, Berkeley.

Campos, P. (2004). *The obesity myth: Why America's obsession with weight is hazardous to your health*. New York: Gotham Books.

Davies, H. T. O., Nutley, S. M., & Smith, P. C. (2000). Introducing evidence-based policy and practice in public services. In T. O. D. Huw, M. N. Sandra, & P. C. Smith (Eds.), *What works? Evidence-based policy and practice in public services*. Bristol: Policy Press.

Davis, G. (2008). 'One big conversation: the Australia 2020 Summit'. *Australian Journal of Public Administration, 67*(4): 379-389.

Dixon, J., & Broom, D. H. (Eds.). (2007). *The seven deadly sins of obesity: How the modern world is making us fat*. Sydney: UNSW Press.

Dunlop, C. (2014). The possible experts: How epistemic communities negotiate barriers to knowledge use in ecosystems services policy. *Environment and Planning C: Government and Policy, 32*(2), 208–228.

Dye, D. T. (2014). New labour, new narrative? Political strategy and the discourse of globalisation. *British Journal of Politics and International Relations, 17*(3), 531–550. doi:10.1111/1467-856X.12043.

Edelman, M. J. (1964). *The symbolic uses of politics*. Urbana, IL: University of Michigan Press.

Egger, G., & Swinburn, B. (2012). *Planet obesity: How we're eating ourselves and the planet to death*. Sydney: Allen and Unwin.

Finlayson, A. (2007). From beliefs to arguments: Interpretive methodology and rhetorical political analysis. *British Journal of Politics and International Relations, 9*(4), 545–563.

Fischer, F. (1995). *Evaluating public policy*. Chicago: Nelson-Hall Publishers.

Fischer, F. (2000). *Citizens, experts, and the environment*. Durham, NC: Duke University Press.

Fischer, F. (2003). *Reframing public policy—Discursive politics and deliberative practices*. Oxford: Oxford University Press.

Fischer, F. (2009). *Democracy and expertise: Reorienting policy inquiry*. Oxford: Oxford University Press.

Fischer, F., & Forester, J. (Eds.). (1993). *The argumentative turn in policy analysis and planning*. Duke, NC: Duke University Press.

Fischer, F., & Gottweis, H. (Eds.). (2012). *The argumentative turn revisited: Public policy as communicative practice*. Duke, NC: Duke University Press.

Flyvbjerg, B. (2006). Five misunderstandings about case-study research. *Qualitative Inquiry, 12*(2), 219–245.

Foresight. (2007). *Tackling obesities: Future choices—Project report (The Foresight Report)*. London: The Stationery Office. Retrieved January 18, 2013, from http://www.bis.gov.uk/assets/foresight/docs/obesity/17.pdf

Freeman, R., & Sturdy, S. (Eds.). (2014). *Knowledge in policy: Embodied, inscribed, enacted*. Bristol: Policy Press.

Gard, M., & Wright, J. (2001). *The obesity epidemic: Science, morality and ideology*. New York: Routledge.

Goffman, E. (1959). *Presentation of self in everday life*. New York: Doubleday.

Gottweis, H. (2007). Rhetoric in policy making. In F. Fischer, G. Miller, & M. Sidney (Eds.), *Handbook of public policy analysis* (pp. 237–250). Boca Raton, FL: CRC Press.

Greenhalgh, T., & Russell, J. (2006). Reframing evidence synthesis as rhetorical action in the policy making drama. *Healthcare Policy, 1*(2), 34–42.

Griggs, S., & Howarth, D. (2013). *The politics of airport expansion in the United Kingdom: Hegemony, policy and the rhetoric of 'sustainable aviation'*. Manchester: Manchester University Press.

Grube, D. (2012). Prime ministers and political narratives for policy change: Towards a heuristic. *Policy and Politics, 40*(4), 569–586.

Hajer, M. A. (2005). Rebuilding ground zero: The politics of performance. *Planning Theory and Practice, 6*(4), 445–464.

Hajer, M. A. (2006). Doing discourse analysis: Coalitions, practices, meaning. In M. van den Brink & T. Metze (Eds.), *Words matter in policy and planning: Discourse theory and method in the social sciences* (pp. 65–74). Utrecht, ND: KNAG/Nethur.

Hajer, M. A. (2009). *Authoritative governance: Policymaking in the age of mediatization*. Oxford: Oxford University Press.

Head, B. (2010). Three lenses of evidence-based policy. *Australian Journal of Public Administration, 67*(1), 1–11.

Hendriks, C. M. (2007). Praxis stories: Experiencing intepretive policy research. *Critical Policy Studies, 1*(3), 278–300.

Hoppe, R. (1999). Policy analysis, science and politics: From "speaking truth to power" to "making sense together". *Science and Public Policy, 26*(3), 201–210.

Hoppe, R. (2010). *The governance of problems. Puzzling, powering, and participation*. Bristol: Policy Press.

House of Representatives (HoR) Standing Committee on Health and Ageing. (2009, February 4). *Inquiry into obesity in Australia*. Canberra: Hansard, Australian Government.

Kelly, J. (2009). What can interdisciplinarity offer to policy problems?: Understanding the public policy of obesity. *European Political Science, 8*(1), 47–56.

Lahsen, M. (2008). Experiences of modernity in the greenhouse: A cultural analysis of a phyisicist "trio" supporting the backlash against global warming. *Global Environmental Change, 18*, 204–219.

Lang, T. (2010, July 21). What a carve up: The coalition is wrong to dismember the Food Standards Agency at the time it is needed most. *The Guardian*. Retrieved January 17, 2013, from http://www.guardian.co.uk/commentis-free/2010/jul/21/fsa-what-a-carve-up

Lang, T., & Rayner, G. (2007). Overcoming policy cacophony on obesity: An ecological public health framework for policymakers. *Obesity Reviews, 8*(Suppl. 1), 165–181.

Lang, T., & Rayner, G. (2012). *Ecological public health: Reshaping the conditions for good health*. London: Routledge.

Lasswell, H. D. (1951). The Policy Orientation. In D. Lerner & H. D. Lasswell (Eds.), *The Policy Sciences* (pp. 3–15). Stanford: Stanford University Press.

Majone, G. (1989). *Evidence, argument and persuasion in the policy process.* New Haven, CT: Yale University Press.

Marmot, M. G. (2004). Evidence-based policy or policy-based evidence? *British Medical Journal, 328,* 906–907.

Monaghan, M. (2011). *Evidence versus politics: Exploiting research in UK drug policy making?* Bristol: Policy Press.

Oliver, J. E. (2005). *Fat politics: The real story behind America's obesity epidemic.* New York: Oxford University Press.

Parsons, W. (2002). From muddling through to muddling up–Evidence based policy making and the modernisation of British government. *Public Policy and Administration, 17*(3), 43–60.

Pawson, R. (2006). *Evidence-based policymaking: A realist critique.* Thousand Oaks, CA: Sage.

Preventative Health Taskforce. (2008). *Technical paper 1—Obesity in Australia: A need for urgent action.* Australian Government, Department of Health and Ageing, Canberra. Retrieved January 21, 2013, from http://www.preventativehealth.org.au/internet/preventativehealth/publishing.nsf/Content/tech-obesity-toc

Preventative Health Taskforce. (2009). *Australia: The healthiest country by 2020.* Australian Government, Department of Health and Ageing, Canberra. Retrieved January 18, 2013, from http://www.preventativehealth.org.au/internet/preventativehealth/publishing.nsf/Content/AEC223A781D64FF0CA2575FD00075DD0/$File/nphs-overview.pdf

Rail, G., Holmes, D., & Murray, S. J. (2010). The politics of evidence on 'domestic terrorists': Obesity discourses and their effects. *Sociological Theory and Health, 8,* 259–279.

Rittel, H. W. J., & Webber, M. (1973). Dilemmas in a general theory of planning. *Policy Sciences, 4,* 155–169.

Roe, E. (1994). *Narrative policy analysis: Theory and practice.* Durham, NC: Duke University Press.

Saguy, A. (2013). *What's wrong with fat?* New York: Oxford University Press.

Schon, D. A. (1983). *The reflective practitioner: How professionals think in action.* London: Temple Smith.

Smith, K. (2013). *Beyond evidence-based policymaking in public health: The interplay of ideas.* Basingstoke: Palgrave Macmillan.

Stone, D. A. (2002). *Policy paradox and political reason: The art of political decision making* (Rev. ed.). New York: W.W. Norton.

Strassheim, H., & Kettunen, P. (2014). When does evidence-based policy turn into policy-based evidence? Configurations, contexts and mechanisms. *Evidence & Policy, 10*(2), 259–277.

Swinburn, B. A., Sacks, G., Hall, K. D., McPherson, K., Finegood, D. T., Moodie, M. L., et al. (2011). The global obesity pandemic: Shaped by global drivers and local environments. *Lancet, 378*(9793), 804–814.

Tenbensel, T. (2006). Policy knowledge for policy work. In H. K. Colebatch (Ed.), *The work of policy: An international survey* (pp. 199–216). Lanham: Lexington Books.

Wang, Y. C., McPherson, K., Marsh, T., Gortmaker, S. L., & Brown, M. (2011). Health and economic burden of the projected obesity trends in the USA and the UK. *Lancet, 378*(9793), 815–825.

Weiss, C. H. (1977). The enlightenment function of social science research. *Policy Analysis, 3*(4), 531–545.

Wesselink, A., & Hoppe, R. (2011). If post-normal science is the solution, what is the problem?: The politics of activist environmental science. *Science Technology and Human Values, 36*, 389–412.

World Health Organization (WHO). (2000). *Obesity: Preventing and managing the global epidemic.* Report of a WHO Consultation, WHO Technical Report Series No. 894, Geneva.

Yanow, D., & Schwartz-Shea, P. (Eds.). (2006). *Interpretation and method: Empirical research methods and the interpretive turn.* New York: ME Sharpe.

Yanow, D., & Schwartz-Shea, P. (2012). *Interpretive research design: Concepts and processes.* New York: Routledge.

Part I

Problem Definition

2

Debating Individual Agency

As discussed in the introductory chapter, obesity is widely regarded as one of the most pressing public health issues of our time. Countless newspaper articles, expert reports, and government inquiries across the world have warned that rising levels of obesity could potentially devastate society as we know it. But beneath this common language of crisis and air of concern lurk different interpretations of what the exact nature of the problem is, who is to blame, and what should be done about it. In recognition of this, scholars in public health, sociology, and political science have paid increasing attention to obesity as a discursively constructed public policy issue.

Within these accounts, the bulk of the focus is on the way the issue has been 'framed' as a problem in the media and in government reports. These studies tend to reduce the discursive battle to a contest over responsibility (e.g. Lawrence 2004; Kim and Anne Willis 2007; Hawkins and Linvill 2010). That is, they tend to present the debate over obesity as informed on the one side with an ideological commitment to collective responsibility for this social problem, and on the other side a commitment to personal responsibility for an individual problem. The particular labels deployed to capture this distinction vary from author to author—some

© The Editor(s) (if applicable) and The Author(s) 2016
J. Boswell, *The Real War on Obesity*,
DOI 10.1057/978-1-137-58252-2_2

refer to the age old 'structure versus agency' divide, others distinguish 'environmental' and 'behavioural' frames or discourses, while others still prefer the language of 'the individual' versus 'the collective'—but what unites them is a stylised representation of a clear dichotomy.[1] While the parsimony presented by such an approach may be useful, especially for the purposes of coding and quantifying debate on obesity in particular sites, it also neglects the complexity of the competing accounts on obesity.

The scholarship on obesity is not unusual in this sense. The bulk of work on the social construction of political and policy problems—especially that subsumed in the 'framing' literature (see van Hulst and Yanow 2014 for a critique)—similarly privileges stylised parsimony over rich nuance. There is a tendency to divide discursive politics into discrete units, with competing frames or discourses taken to engender completely different views of the world (or acknowledge completely different ontologies). Of course, the appeal and use of such analytic neatness is obvious. Social science is at heart a task of providing simplified heuristics to aid understanding of exceptionally complex phenomena. But, I will argue here, something is also lost, and there are benefits from acknowledging and understanding overlaps and intersections that mitigate the prospect of discrete, coherent constructions of complex issues. Certainly, most of the narratives I identify in this analysis, at least in the hands of some proponents, bridge any rigidly imposed 'frames' or 'discourses' at that level of abstraction; far more happens in political debate than any simple manifestation of the structure versus agency or individual versus collective binary.

Indeed, what I hope to show in this chapter is that the primary debate about obesity as a policy issue in Australia and in the UK centres not around whether obesity is at heart an environmental or behavioural issue, but about the 'mix' of these contributing factors. The contest is about the degree of emphasis that ought to be placed on the individual vis-à-vis the

---

[1] There are of course some important exceptions. Barry et al. (2009), for instance, acknowledge a broader variety of constructions in their account of the 'metaphors' that order policymakers ideas and preferences on obesity. Swierstra (2011) likewise makes room for a more complex array of obesity 'discourses'. And most valuably of all, Shugart (2011) develops a sophisticated analysis of the now dominant sociological narrative of obesity, in which she consciously undermines the typical 'environmental versus behavioural' divide. This analysis builds on this work, especially that of Shugart, in the task of unpacking a more nuanced political debate about obesity as a policy issue.

collective, and thus what policy instruments are best placed to deal with the issue of rapidly rising obesity. Proponents of the two most prominent narratives on obesity in both cases—using Roe's (1994) terminology, the 'dominant' account that largely orders official policy in both countries and the primary 'counternarrative' that underpins the most vociferous and broadest opposition to this status quo—both draw on broader environmental and behavioural discourses about the issue. The key distinction here is that they mobilise them in different ways, and to different degrees, to promote and underpin different accounts of the issue that lead to different policy solutions. These findings have important implications for work on the social construction of policy issues, promoting a narrative approach that can uncover the drama of policy debate as it unfolds across sites of debate and over time. They also pave the way for a much more nuanced account of the discursive politics of obesity. As importantly, in the context of this book, they provide the background against which the following chapters, outlining more marginal or oppositional narratives, can be understood.

I start by briefly contextualising my narrative approach within the broader field of the social construction of complex policy problems. I then outline the dominant narrative—Facilitated Agency—before recounting its primary counter—Structured Opportunity. I highlight the 'mix' of environmental/structure and behavioural/agency apparent in each, before considering the implications both for further work on social construction of policy problems (including obesity) and for the analysis to come.

Defining Policy Problems: The Narration of Obesity

Work on the social construction of policy problems is now very much mainstream. There is a widespread understanding that policy problems are not given; their importance, nature, meaning, and resolution are socially constructed. Defining problems is political. Indeed, arguably the bulk of the focus in contemporary policy studies is on the way in which actors fight to get their issue on the agenda and then, once there, fight to make their understanding of the issue the dominant understanding. There is a vast and growing literature on 'framing', in particular, that attempts to capture these dynamics in action (see Chong and Druckman 2007 for a review). This is not to simplistically promote a narrative approach at the expense of a framing one. Much of the most active scholarship on narrative focuses similarly on given texts and their impact in political settings (see Jones and McBeth 2007; Shenhav 2005, 2006; Sheafer et al. 2011).

Regardless of the particular label deployed, in practice the task of the analyst in such work is to identify dichotomous frames (or narratives) around which conflict revolves—indeed, there are usually just two—and then assign components of the relevant text under analysis into each category in order to make claims about (and typically quantify) the relative strength of frames. This is precisely the case with much of the most influential work on the construction of obesity, which reduces its politics to a simple contest between environment and behaviour. There are obvious advantages and appeals to such analysis but, as van Hulst and Yanow (2014) explain, they are limited by their static or rigid representation of discursive politics.

More surprisingly, rival work on *discourse* suffers from similar limitations in practice. This is surprising because scholars who use this term typically espouse a constructivist epistemology and aim to be sensitive to contextual meaning. Understood as 'an ensemble of ideas, concepts, and categories through which meaning is given to social and physical phenomena' (Hajer 1995, p. 63), discourses emerge as distinctive sets of ideas and claims about what exists and what matters in a relevant policy field (see Dryzek 1996). What this means is that discourse analyses have potential to reveal a greater variety of interpretations than dichotomous framing analyses. But discourse analysts tend to place particular emphasis on distinct ontological beliefs that define divergent discourses (see, e.g. Dryzek 1996, Chap. 2). In practice, this means that such analyses tend again to be rigid in their categorisations of contestation over meaning. The point remains that actors do not talk or think about the issue in such categorical terms.

To be very clear, my aim here is not to denigrate discourse as an analytical tool. Discourse analysts do a vital job of identifying and bringing forth the background assumptions that underpin the way actors make sense of and argue about policy issues, and I make reference to some of these in the discussion that follows. But political actors seldom speak coherently and discretely within discourses. Indeed, discourse analysts themselves acknowledge discourses do not necessarily map onto the way that actors think and talk about complex political problems in practice (see Hajer 1995; Szarka 2004). And so relevant work on obesity sheds important light on the discourses that condition debate on obesity— Swierstra (2011), for instance, usefully sets the environmental and behavioural against the biomedical and social as well. But, as I will show, actors typically bridge or mix these rigid categories in their espoused interpretation of the issue.

As such, I favour a narrative approach that, I suggest, better captures the dramatic contest over meaning as it unfolds in political debate. Such an approach can marry parsimony with nuance, allowing the analyst to appreciate the intersections, overlaps, and grey areas of political debate. It focuses on how actors can cross-reference experiences, beliefs, and assumptions associated with divergent frames or discourses in working to make sense of complex information and convince other actors of their cause.[2] Inspired in particular by the works of Roe (1994) and Stone (2002), I show how actors not only work to draw on but also reconcile apparently distinct 'frames' or 'discourses' in their efforts to narrate in practice.

Specifically, my recounting of each narrative begins with a broad plot summary which outlines the starting point of the narrative, the problem as it develops, the current or impending crisis that it leads to, and the heroic intervention required to save the day. Embedded within each account is a breakdown of the key characters thought to play an important role in moving the plot along, and a discussion of the key symbols and slogans associated with the narrative. In recognition of the point laboured throughout the book so far that narratives are not dead texts but live acts,

---

[2] Elsewhere I have drawn out the analytical distinction between narrative and discourse (see Boswell 2013). The key point for the purposes of this discussion is that narratives represent how actors reflexively think and talk about issues, where discourses represent constellations of ideas that, though seldom recounted in full, order people's perspectives on understanding of political issues, sometimes at a distance from or beyond their own apprehension.

I also look at how these competing accounts are typically performed in key policy settings (though Part 2 will present a more detailed analysis of how, and to what effect, they can be performed differently in distinct sites).

Of course, before outlining this analysis, it is important to mention at the outset a couple of caveats. One is that while areas of fuzziness and overlap in the interplay between these narratives (and indeed the ones recounted in subsequent chapters) become a particular feature of my analysis in Part 2 of the book, in Part 1 and in this chapter in particular my aim is to achieve clarity for the reader and present these as distinct accounts. Two is that although the narratives that emerge from the full wealth of data are immensely rich and intricately detailed—especially in comparison with much of the existing work on the social construction of obesity—inevitably my representation of them here is also somewhat pared back or stylised. Such are the trade-offs of conducting and writing up interpretive research (see Boswell and Corbett 2015). The risk is, of course, that I open myself up to precisely the same critique I have made of the existing framing literature, although I still contend that my analysis provides a richer, deeper, and more nuanced account than what already exists in the literature on obesity, or often elsewhere. I have endeavoured to recreate the narratives here in a way that lends plenty of colour and context to them, while still allowing space for deeper analytical examination of the impact on debate and policy work, especially as explored in Part 2 of the book.

With that background in mind, I move on to outline the competing narratives that comprise the 'main debate' in both countries. Both, as I will show, bridge the rigid frames typically imposed in analyses of the social construction of this issue.

Narrative 1: Facilitated Agency

The Facilitated Agency narrative is 'dominant' in both Australia and the UK in the sense that it receives support from the broadest coalition, including most of the influential decision-makers. It is also the narrative that, in most cases, underpins official government policies in both Australia and the UK. This narrative holds that rising obesity rates are symptomatic of changes in society, and that people need help in reconnecting to healthier lifestyles (Text Box 2.1). It is perhaps best summed up by former Australian Minister of Health and Ageing, Nicola Roxon:

> Losing weight doesn't have to be hard: those little decisions made in the supermarket aisles, in the kitchen or when playing with the kids, can make a real difference. (Quoted in Wright 2011)

Text Box 2.1

Facilitated Agency

Essence
Social changes have driven obesity because individuals have lost touch with healthy lifestyles.

Main proponents
Food industry, politicians, bureaucrats, some experts, celebrities

Characters
Villains: Social changes
Victims: Obese people
Heroes: Committed 'stakeholders'

Targets of intervention
Consumers through education

Symbols and slogans
- 'We're all in this together.'
- 'Not nannying, but nudging'

Performance
- Diffuse—sometimes defensive, enthusiastic, or sombre

In both Australia and the UK, this narrative starts with a nostalgic view of the past. A generation or two ago, it is thought, people were overwhelmingly of a healthy weight. They enjoyed a well-proportioned diet of home-cooking and 'did not have any of that take-away stuff' (Liberals MP M May in HoR Inquiry, November 26, 2008g, p. 7). Moreover, they were physically fit both because they sought recreation outdoors and because most worked in an environment conducive to incidental exercise. Mark Coulton, a Nationals MP in the House of Representatives and a member of the Health and Ageing Committee which conducted the HoR Inquiry on Obesity opined:

> When I left school 30 years ago, my friends in the footy team were timber workers, farmers, shearers and electricity workers. Those electricity workers went up and down a ladder 20 times a day ... All they needed were two runs around the oval and a drink of water to be ready for the footy season. (HoR Inquiry, September 11, 2008c, p. 75)

Major changes in the make-up of society are seen as disrupting this healthy way of life. It is assumed that since the secure family unit, with a mother's primary role in the home, has given way to a whole new range of family dynamics, families have become time poor, and as a consequence people often lack basic food preparation skills. This point was clearly encapsulated in an interview with renowned author, Barbara Kingsolver: '[My generation of women] lost a lot—we traded our aprons for the min-ivan and the Lunchable, and the result was children with health problems because we pick up junk food on the way to the soccer game' (quoted in Pilkington 2008).

Under this narrative, technological advancements are also seen to have changed people's lifestyles. It is thought that many people, especially chil-dren, have taken to entertaining themselves through playing computer games, watching television, or surfing the Internet rather than through outdoor pursuits. This situation is thought to be further perpetuated by widespread concerns about safety, which preclude opportunities for inci-dental exercise and play. Former English football star Michael Owen said in an interview:

> When I was young, my mum was quite happy to let me go outdoors on my own but she'd think twice about it now because the streets are no longer as safe. I certainly wouldn't be keen to let my kids go to the park on their own. (Quoted in Crace 2008)

The Facilitated Agency narrative also takes into account changes in working life. Children are thought not to get the life coaching they need at school, with priority placed on other parts of an ever-expanding curriculum rather than the value of educating young people about physical education and home economics. One expert witness at an HoR hearing explained: 'I look to ask the schools one more time to do more when I know we are not paying teachers enough to do everything else' (HoR Inquiry, December 8, 2008i, p. 16.). It is also suggested that most modern workplaces require employees to be seated and inactive for longer, robbing them of time that could be spent exercising afterwards as well as contributing to poor dietary choices (interview with a British health official, June 2012).

To compound matters, it is thought that people do not just lack the time and skills to maintain a healthy lifestyle, but awareness about its importance. Proponents of this narrative argue that ordinary people, parents in particular, have become confused by a cacophony of expert (and commercial) messages about exercise and food. Lacking the experiential grounding enjoyed by older generations to help make sense of it all, these people are assumed to have lost touch with what constitutes a healthy lifestyle. A *Sun Herald* journalist concluded:

> Public health initiatives prompted by the initial spike in childhood obesity levels in the 1980s and '90s resulted in a flurry of rules around both 'good' and 'bad' foods. These, combined with often conflicting messages flooding out of the diet, wellness and self-help industries, left some parents feeling adrift in a sea of information. (Lewis 2011)

Indeed, the rot is thought to have set in to such an extent that people no longer even understand what is healthy and what is not. An expert commented at an HoR hearing that the majority of parents of obese children do not recognise the fact, and that only a fraction of those who do even see it as a problem (HoR Inquiry, June 13, 2008a, p. 29).

The heroic intervention prescribed in this narrative is to cut through this quagmire by clarifying the message, encouraging people to re-embrace healthy eating and physical activity. The goal of public policy in relation to this issue should be to raise awareness of the problem right across the community, provide people with the skills they need to succeed in losing and keeping off weight, offer incentives for them to lead healthy lifestyles, and empower them in their pursuit of these goals. The suggestion is that creating such an environment will result in individuals assuming greater control over their decision-making and thus deriving significant health benefits. An editorial for an Australian tabloid surmised:

> The key to curbing obesity is with parents and their children. Parents need to be educated about their children's nutritional needs to nip unhealthy eating habits before they take hold. If we don't rethink what's on the dinner table tonight, we're looking at a future of increased diabetes, cardiovascular disease, osteoarthritis and some cancers. Now that's really hard to stomach. (*The Sun Herald* 2008b)

In order to get there, importantly, it is assumed that there are limits to what government can actually achieve. UK Minister of the Cabinet Office Francis Maude (2010) expressed this in a column for the *Guardian*, arguing that 'legislation has its limitations' and that in policy areas like healthcare 'the government has thrown huge sums of money at problems with limited success'. Indeed, in the UK in recent times, the Facilitated Agency narrative has become associated with behavioural economics, or so-called 'nudge theory', and the notion that government policy is dependent on utilising individual agency. Based on social science theory and research, the belief is that people's behaviour can be subtly 'nudged' by establishing appropriate incentives and default settings (see Thaler and Sunstein 2008). Secretary of State Andrew Lansley suggested when he publicly unveiled the government's new public health policy agenda:

> It is time for politicians to stop telling people to make health choices, time for them to start helping them to do it. We are not nannying, but nudging. (Quoted in White 2010)

Likewise, potential heroes beyond the state and the individual are seen as having key roles to play, too. The food industry, in particular, is thought to be crucial in self-regulating the marketing and labelling of unhealthy products, and reformulating them to be healthier in the first place (interview with an Australian food industry representative,

May 2011; interview with a British clinician, May 2012). Individuals, parents, and communities are expected to take responsibility for their own health, too. As such, the slogan that best encapsulates this narrative is that 'we're all in this together'[3]: the prevailing perception is that all of the characters involved in this narrative are seen to have a degree of agency; all have contributed to the problem, and all can contribute to the solution.

Performing the Facilitated Agency Narrative

This narrative has the most diverse range of adherents, including some academics and practitioners, some NGO representatives, some media commentators, and most politicians, bureaucrats, community leaders, food industry representatives, weight loss and fitness industry representatives and their 'success stories', and a handful of celebrity activists. As well as being performed by different actors, the Facilitated Agency narrative is also performed in very different ways.

Backstage, some actors aggressively lobby decision-makers and media outlets, while others (or at different times the same actors) are more magnanimous in both their formal correspondence and informal networking. In the UK, for instance, adherents to the Facilitated Agency narrative have attempted to influence the deliberations of the Food Standards Agency (FSA) board on obesity-related issues like nutrient profiling and product labelling. For some, this has meant a commitment to positive engagement with the board. The Department of Health—whose members have mainly performed and reinforced the Facilitated Agency narrative—regularly updates the board on strategic developments and policy planning. Others, though, have taken a more adversarial stance to what they perceive as the board's political agenda, aggressively challenging their processes. This has manifested in lobbying of the media to portray the FSA in an unflattering light, and more direct efforts to influence the

---

[3] This was the tagline of the Public Health Commission in the UK—a forerunner to the current Responsibility Deals that was established by the Conservative party while in opposition. For a lengthy commentary, see Lawrence (2010).

board's deliberations by protesting about aspects of the agenda for particular meetings.[4]

Likewise, in the front stage, the Facilitated Agency narrative is performed with everything from an infectious energy through celebrity adherents to a staid objectivity by health bureaucrats. One example of how diffuse this support can be was showcased through the performances of the committee members in the HoR Inquiry in Australia. All performed the Facilitated Agency account, but the way they articulated and enacted it during the course of the Inquiry differed greatly. Liberals MPs Jamie Briggs and Margaret May at times took an adversarial stance to the expert witnesses they met with. Briggs, for instance, interrupted one expert to question his simplistic vilification of junk food (HoR, Perth hearing, 2008, pp. 21–22), and taunted another after a testy interaction that he 'might go to McDonald's for lunch' (HoR, Melbourne, 2008, p. 51). In contrast, other committee members like Mark Coulton of The Nationals and Jill Hall of Labor tended to align themselves with these experts—they responded warmly and earnestly to the experts' testimony, and certainly did not challenge it. But their broader account of obesity, and their support for the recommendations of the HoR Inquiry, remained the same.

Narrative 2: Structured Opportunity

The Structured Opportunity narrative is the primary counter to the dominant Facilitated Agency account. It is the one that majority of public health experts and academics across Australia and the UK put forward, suggesting that the rise in rates of obesity is an alarming and potentially destructive consequence of a skewed marketplace. This is seen to have created a 'toxic' or 'obesogenic' environment which in equal part feeds on and further inhibits individual or behavioural weaknesses in respect to food consumption and rates of physical activity. The essence of this narrative is that individuals are struggling to adapt to the physical and especially food environment they now find themselves in, and that

---

[4] For example, the Food and Drink Federation corresponded with board members the day before a meeting on April 10, 2008, to voice grave concerns about the proposed agenda.

strong-armed government intervention is required to regulate the food market in particular and develop structures that better support informed consumer choice (Text Box 2.2).

Text Box 2.2

Structured Opportunity

Essence
The obesity crisis is a consequence of individual vulnerability to industry excess and a lack of regulation.

Main proponents
Public health experts, left-wing commentators

Characters and causation
Villains: Big Food
Victims: Consumers
Heroes: Public health experts

Symbols and slogans
- The 'toxic' environment
- An obesity 'epidemic'

Targets of intervention
The food industry

Performance
- Urgent
- Frustrated
- Deliberately concerted

As with the Facilitated Agency narrative, this account begins with a nostalgic view of eating and exercise habits decades ago. The suggestion is that people used to be healthy primarily because they had control over what they ate. In both countries, this happy equilibrium is seen to have been undermined by faults in the broader social and economic structures in which food consumption choices are made—faults that are at least in part the result of the undermining actions of private interests. The primary villain is Big Food—the fast food restaurant industry as well as processed food manufacturers and retailers. They are seen to have insidiously designed, manufactured, and promoted their products to maximise profits at the expense of public health. A journalist from the *Age* suggested:

> Not so long ago, it was easy to tell which foods were good for you and which were not—what was a staple, what was a treat. Now, it is less clear. And public health advocates will tell you, that is no accident; it is the result of clever marketing strategies by the powerful food industry. (Williams 2011)

Perhaps worse still, Big Food is seen to be meddling in the political process to avoid the firm regulation that proponents of this narrative claim is so badly needed. Recent efforts to paint themselves as 'part of the solution' and to appear to be engaging in voluntary initiatives around marketing, labelling, and product reformulation are dismissed as 'weight-wash' (interview with an Australian public health advocate, June 2011; interview with a British clinician, April 2012). Furthermore, some proponents of this narrative accuse Big Food of having covered their actions up by deliberately muddying the evidence around obesity and the marketing and sale of unhealthy food. Jane Martin, the spokesperson for public health lobby group the Obesity Policy Coalition and outspoken advocate of this narrative in Australia, asked:

> Where's the honesty? That's exactly what the tobacco industry did, they debated whether smoking was addictive and caused a whole lot of confusion … We used to have cigarettes sold with diaries, with CDs and key rings. Now we've got fast food sold with toys and movie tie-ins. They argue it's not there to encourage consumption—so why do they do it? (Quoted in Stark 2009a)

But Big Food is not the only villainous industry in this portrayal. Car manufacturers are depicted as conspiring with property developers, urban planners, and engineers to ensure that the primary objective of urban design is gaining convenient access for cars rather than promoting healthy and sustainable lifestyles (interview with Australian planning expert, June 2011). The fitness and weight loss industries, too, are seen to have seized on the rising levels of overweight and obesity as a money-making opportunity. This is a point only reinforced by recent commercial tie-ups between food manufacturers such as Nestle and weight loss companies such as Jenny Craig. Jane Martin, again, has been an outspoken critic on this point:

What we're seeing is the careful execution of strategies by processed food manufacturers to ensure a long-term future. They're broadening their coverage by selling consumers the problem and then also being on hand to sell them the solution. (Quoted in Stark 2011)

In light of this, recent government efforts to improve awareness of healthy lifestyles are seen as hopeless. On the Australian government's refusal to legislate on 'junk food' advertising, journalist Adelle Horin (2008) argued that 'education can't on its own compete with the massive advertising dollar of the junk food industry'. It is felt that the conviction needed to go beyond these superficial actions and implement effective, population-wide policy is lacking due to fear of the ramifications from the powerful food industry. In response to the announcement of the Responsibility Deal approach to public health, a *Guardian* columnist exclaimed:

[The] revelation that fast food and drinks companies such as McDonald's, PepsiCo, Unilever and Diageo have now been asked by ministers to draw up public health policy shows the corporate takeover of politics has reached a new level. This isn't an issue of government consulting business. We're talking about the same vested interests that have fuelled the obesity and alcohol abuse crises as good as dictating terms at the heart of government. (Milne 2010)

This situation is thought to have been exacerbated by excessive focus on treatment or finding a miracle cure. Indeed, there is an especially strong distrust of the pharmaceutical industry and its efforts to establish a 'cure' for obesity. A recurrent joke a number of my interview participants—especially those who support the Structured Opportunity account—made was that the obesity 'wonderdrug' is always 10 years away from mass production, even in 10 years' time. But there is a serious point to this concern. The high-profile nature of medical research is seen to draw funding away from crucial areas of research on population-wide measures, and, perhaps more importantly, provide a (probably) false hope which props up the unsustainable system of food production and consumption (interview with a British public health advocate, January 2012). In the pursuit of this mythical 'magic bullet', it is thought that the experience and expertise of the key heroes in this narrative—public health experts—remain unappreciated or forgotten. Many bemoaned the pitiful funding given to prevention as compared to acute services. This was, for them, the ambulance at the bottom of the cliff.

Overall, the actions of various industries and the relative inaction of government are thought to have resulted in skyrocketing rates of obesity. Proponents of this narrative believe that ordinary people have become stuck in a 'candy shop' of temptation. One expert witness at the HoR Inquiry summed it up:

> our way of life has become very sedentary and our foods have become very energy dense. If you look at our society, it is almost a normal reaction for people, children and adults, to gain weight inappropriately. (HoR Inquiry, September 11, 2008c, p. 72)

With skyrocketing rates of obesity comes an 'epidemic' or 'tsunami' of lifestyle-related chronic illness (interview with an Australian public health expert, June 2011). The notion is that rising obesity rates have already put increasing pressure on public hospitals and, as the situation deteriorates in the future, it will jeopardise the long-term sustainability of the health service. In a letter to the *Guardian*, a spokesperson for the British Medical Association voiced concern about the future of Britain's iconic National Health Service (NHS):

> The UK is facing an obesity crisis and there are already around 1 million obese children under 16 …. While there is no precise figure for how much obesity costs the NHS, we know that every year it spends at least £2 billion on treating ill-health caused by unhealthy diets. (V Nathanson in the *Guardian* 2010)

The same is thought to be true of Medicare in Australia, where public health expert Paul Zimmet has been even more forthright: 'This is the biggest public health problem Australia has ever faced and if we can't turn it around, we'll have a situation where we'll almost bankrupt the health systems of this nation' (quoted in Stark 2008).

The heroic intervention in this narrative is for brave and urgent government action in adopting a strong-armed approach towards protecting the interests of consumers. The direct target of public policy in this account ought to be the food industry. The solution, it is suggested, should involve imposing a suite of regulations, including clamping down on advertising and marketing of unhealthy food (especially to children), improving labelling for consumers, changing subsidies around food production and tax incentives at point of sale, instigating changes in planning policy, careful monitoring of diet and exercise programs, and generally making obesity prevention a major, cross-sectoral government priority. The emphasis must be on regulating at the population-wide level, rather than through pressuring individuals to make lifestyle changes in the face of overwhelming temptation. The point is made forcefully by renowned Australian public health expert Simon Chapman (2009):

> The frightening speed with which obesity is increasing globally requires bold policy. The obesity epidemic will not be stalled or reversed by cosmetic initiatives like small community health promotion campaigns, but by policy reforms that reach every Australian.

Performing the Structured Opportunity Narrative

The Structured Opportunity account is an expert-dominated account, performed largely by public health researchers and practitioners behind, in and across the various sites of deliberation. Just as significant as this uniformity of cast is the fact that the actors tend to narrate it in very similar ways. This is not to suggest that they always refer to the same images and evidence in their accounts. In fact, one proponent of the Structured Opportunity narrative explained that the opposite was the case—that her 'message was pitched' specifically for the audience (interview with an Australian primary health advocate, June 2011). However, their performances almost always serve to convey a seriousness about the scale of the problem, a strong sense of urgency about the need for action, and a frustration about the perceived barriers to implementing an effective plan.

The impression of a concerted, coordinated coalition is no accident, either; in fact it represents a conscious strategy on the part of the narrative's leading proponents. Borne partly out of resentment of the perceived power of the food industry to influence policy, and partly out of fears over the damaging impact of 'policy cacophony' and a lack of clarity for decision-makers (see Lang and Rayner 2007), these actors have consciously banded together to form a more united voice. Their belief is that in doing so they will have greater influence:

> And the way we've attempted to strengthen our hands is to make sure that we are working with those other groups. Because our chances of getting better outcomes are always enhanced no end when we have a series of health groups that are involved. (Interview with an Australian public health advocate, April 2011)

Backstage, actors who subscribe to this narrative have apparently harried decision-makers and journalists to try to get them to appreciate the urgency of the matter. Indeed, one Australian politician repeatedly used the word 'zealot' in our interview to describe the most vocal public health advocates she deals with (interview with an Australian Senator, May 2011). For example, the movement for an Inquiry on protecting children from 'junk food' advertising in Australia came on the back of concerted lobbying. The heavy emphasis on this particular issue was thought by proponents of Structured Opportunity to represent a 'strategic low-hanging fruit' that might galvanise support for their wider claims (interview with an Australian clinician, June 2011). These actors brought pressure to bear on policymakers by stressing the urgency of the situation and giving the impression of political support for their cause. As one politician involved in the process explained:

> there was an amazing email campaign around the country saying, 'We've got to stop junk food advertising'. It touches a button with people, particularly parents out in the network. (Interview with an Australian Senator, May 2011)

This sense of urgency and frustration is also conveyed through the enactment of the narrative in different sites front stage. This was nowhere better exemplified than at the very same Inquiry, where a long list of experts lined up to voice support for Bob Brown's bill. The most striking presentation was a combined effort from six advocates from various health NGOs, public research, and health professional organisations. This panel outnumbered the committee members by a ratio of two-to-one, and inundated them with wave after wave of almost identical testimony. The effect was a relentless enactment of Structured Reform, reinforcing the urgency and seriousness of the cause.

Structure Versus Agency? 'Making Healthy Choices Easier'

Readers may still, at this juncture, question whether the account adds anything new to what is already known about the social construction of obesity. At a quick glance, what I call the Facilitated Agency and Structured Opportunity narratives may seem to correspond more or less to the environmental versus behavioural or individual versus collective dichotomies that I began this chapter by critiquing. Yet in fact what I have attempted to foreshadow in my stylised recounting of these narratives, and will now tease out in greater depth and clarity, is the way in which both borrow from the same set of discourses; they bring together, in different 'mixes' and in different manners, aspects of the broader environmental and behavioural explanation for rising obesity, and aspects of the broader individual and collective representations of how the problem might best be solved.

This was a point made clear to me in an exchange with my very first interview participant. I asked this Australian NGO representative—and firm advocate of the Structured Opportunity account—why, in all my documentary analysis, I had not come across any actor who conveyed a purely 'behavioural' account of obesity in formal or elite spaces of democracy. He replied:

There's two parts to the policy. They're really at opposite ends of the spectrum. One's the personal responsibility element about your own personal

fitness—your own personal diet and nutrition. And by and large governments have been quite good in running campaigns that encourage personal
fitness, encourage personal responsibility. But in fact there are a huge
number of structural issues. And that's the other side of the debate. There
are a huge number of structural issues that also need government's attention. So the Tony Abbotts (then Opposition Health Spokesperson), the
Kate Carnells (then Food and Grocery Council representative) of the world
like to emphasise—they recognise the structural issues—but they emphasise the personal responsibility. I suppose if I was putting a percentage on it
I'd say the personal responsibility element is 20% and the structural issues
are 80%. It's a bit hard to put a percentage on it. But you know I'm just
trying to give you an indication of the sort of emphasis. [Abbott and
Carnell] would put the emphasis around the other way.

This was also something that proponents of the Facilitated Agency
account were also more than willing to concede. In response to a query
challenging his defence of the Facilitated Agency narrative in comparison
to the widespread support for the Structured Opportunity narrative among
many of his friends and former colleagues, one official (and ex-academic)
pushed back in our interview. Cognisant of the literature on the environmental versus behavioural construction of obesity, he asserted that in his
opinion obesity should be best defined and understood as a confluence of
environmental and behavioural factors. He summed the point up as follows:

But it isn't just a matter of stupidity or laziness and so on. The easy option
is one that humans tend to take in the way we live and eat and think and
so on. None of that can diminish the fact that walk down a typical high
street centre anywhere in the UK and you can get plentiful calories quickly,
cheaply, easily, and people therefore do. When you think of that, you know,
big changes in the way we live our lives, the way we travel, the way we
work, along with an environment which is packed with easy options, and
on top of that, with human behaviour being what it is, we will tend to take
the easier options put in front of us. (Interview with a British public health
official, June 2012)

But nowhere was this invocation of a 'mix' more clearly spelled out
than in the discursive contest over a key slogan. At the core, proponents

of both the dominant Facilitated Agency narrative and the Structured Opportunity counternarrative claimed to be 'making healthy choices easier'.[5] Proponents of the Facilitated Agency account hope to achieve this by taking steps (both on the part of government and in conjunction with partners in industry and the third sector) to educate and enlighten consumers. Their story is that arming people with such knowledge will effectively empower them to make better choices about nutrition and exercise. For proponents of the Structured Opportunity account, in contrast, 'making healthy choices easier' revolves more around removing distractions and distortions that currently work to confuse people. They want a fairer or more open marketplace in which consumers can better exercise their judgement. Crucially, though, for both success in 'making healthy choices easier' depends inevitably on the exercise of both individual and collective action. Indeed, at times it was striking just how similar proponents of rival narratives, who pressed for very different policy outcomes and often expressed intense animosity towards one another at a personal and professional level, could actually sound.

Take this example from opinion columns submitted to an Australian daily in relatively quick succession. In the first, a clear advocate of the Structured Opportunity account claimed:

> Everyone—individuals, families, schools, workplaces, communities, media, health services, industry and all tiers and sectors of government— will need to take responsibility if we are to turn around the current obesity trend. Unfortunately there is no quick or easy fix. The magnitude of the solution needs to match the magnitude of the problem. (Johnson 2010)

The second, weeks later from Australia's chief food industry advocate, Kate Carnell (2010)—key narrator of Facilitated Agency and self-confessed 'enemy number 1' of most public health experts and practitioners—uses almost the exact same wording:

---

[5] This was the tagline of an influential Cabinet Office White Paper in 2004, promoted and referred to often by advocates of the Facilitated Agency account, especially in Britain. It was also adopted as an important subheading in the report of the National Preventative Health Taskforce (2008)— considered a key articulation of the Structured Opportunity narrative in Australia.

There is no quick fix for the growing levels of obesity. We will reverse the trend only with a comprehensive partnership approach involving governments, business, community and individual responsibility for our personal health and our families.

Conclusion

Clearly, then, to proponents of both the dominant narratives in Australia and Britain's obesity debate, the story of obesity ultimately involves a 'mix' of environmental and behavioural factors, and its satisfactory denouement depends on the exercise of both collective and individual responsibility in some combination. The nature of this 'mix', or the ratio of ingredients within it, remains quite different, and in fact represents the primary point of contention across these two narratives[6]; yet the point remains that proponents of the Facilitated Agency and Structured Opportunity accounts have sought to mobilise greater support by telling narratives that 'bridge' broader discourses of the issue.

Looking beyond the significance for the case of obesity and relevant scholarship therein, there are important parallels in this finding with Dryzek's (2010) recent account of rhetoric in democratic deliberation. Though Dryzek's account is primarily a normative one, he draws on the language of social capital theory to identify the potential empirically for 'bridging' and 'bonding' rhetoric—the former being the use of language to appeal to fellow adherents of a given discourse and the latter being the use of language to appeal to, and try to persuade, adherents of a rival discourse. He provides a brief empirical vignette, in the form of Martin Luther King's historic 'I Have a Dream' speech, as an example of (in his account, normatively desirable) 'bridging rhetoric'. The evidence presented in this chapter provides a much fuller empirical examination of this

---

[6] Interestingly, the nature of the 'mix' can also vary greatly across performances of the same narrative in different settings of debate. Namely, relative to their accounts in expert-dominated sites or in the media, advocates of the key counternarrative are more likely to downplay aspects of the 'environmental' discourse and emphasise aspects of the 'behavioural' discourse on obesity when engaging with policymakers in decision-oriented sites of discussion and policy work. I will return to this point in depth in subsequent chapters, especially in Part 2 of the book, as the theme of fuzziness and disjuncture across debate emerges more clearly.

phenomenon: it shows how actors narrate in practice in ways that draw across rival and seemingly incompatible discourses. The effect, leaving aside any (and perhaps debatable) normative benefits, and even regardless of whether it is a conscious advocacy strategy on their part or not, is to enhance the appeal of their preferred narrative across a broader audience.

Such a finding should therefore be of key interest to scholars of policy narratives, or more generally of the social construction of public problems. It lends a more nuanced hue to an area of scholarship often characterised by parsimonious, dichotomous representations—a state of affairs I have argued is especially the case in relation to the relevant literature on obesity. But this is not to say that the tendency towards the complex 'bridging' that occurs in both Australia and the UK in this analysis always occurs. Nor is it to say that it is always profitable for those seeking to influence policy even if it does. Important further work is needed to assess in what ways, or if at all, the findings made in this case comparison resonate with work across other policy domains and regions.

As well as providing a fine-grained account of the 'main debate' on obesity which should resonate more broadly across discussion of complex and contested policy issues, another important aspect of this analysis is that it uncovers important narratives further towards the margins of debate. In particular, given the overall aims of the book to better understand the ways in which knowledge is interpreted and used in policy debate and policy work, a standout feature is that many of the 'experts' engaged in debate do not subscribe to either of the dominant pair of narratives. Instead, my analysis identifies two rival expert accounts that sit uncomfortably behind, and alongside, the dominant narrative and counternarrative described in this chapter.

The defining characteristic in this dominant pair of narratives, and the theme running through this chapter, has been a focus on the question of agency. The pair in the next chapter deal with this question as well—indeed, any attempt to make sense of a significant problem in public life inevitably bumps up against it—but the discrepancy is better understood and outlined as a debate about the scope of the issue. The Facilitated Agency and Structured Opportunity narratives share more or less similar horizons, with obesity represented as a problem associated with an imbalance in consumption and exertion, and its solution ultimately in working to redress the balance through a mix of regulation and nudging. In contrast, the expert accounts offered in the next section represent interpretations of obesity that greatly shrink or expand the scope of the problem, and thus the nature of the required policy response. I turn my attention to this distinction, and its implications, now.

References

Barry, C. L., Brescoll, V. L., Brownell, K. D., & Schlesinger, M. (2009). Obesity metaphors: How beliefs about the causes of obesity affect support for public policy. *Milbank Quarterly, 87*(1), 7–47.

Boswell, J. (2013). Why and how narrative matters in deliberative systems. *Political Studies, 61*(3), 620–636.

Boswell, J., & Corbett, J. (2015). Embracing impressionism: Revealing the brush strokes of interpretive research. *Critical Policy Studies, 9*(2), 216–225.

Carnell, K. (2010, November 13). Should junk food advertising to kids be banned? *The Sydney Morning Herald.* Retrieved January 15, 2013, from http://newsstore.fairfax.com.au/apps/viewDocument.ac;jsessionid=2D03B5 419AAA3FE571C5F0236242297D?sy=afr&pb=all_ffx&dt=selectRange&d r=1month&so=relevance&sf=text&sf=headline&rc=10&rm=200&sp=brs& cls=7&clsPage=1&docID=SMH1011131K2N3D137LP

Chapman, S. (2009, September 2). Prevention: A track record to die for. *The Sydney Morning Herald.* Retrieved January 15, 2013, from http://www.smh.com.au/opinion/contributors/prevention-a-track-record-to-die-for-20090901-f6ub.html

Chong, D., & Druckman, J. N. (2007). Framing theory. *Annual Review of Political Science, 10*, 103–126.

Crace, J. (2008, March 4). A healthy debate. *The Guardian.* Retrieved January 15, 2013, from http://www.guardian.co.uk/education/2008/mar/04/school-sports.schools

Dryzek, J. S. (1996). *The politics of the earth: Environmental discourses.* New York: Oxford University Press.

Dryzek, J. S. (2010). Rhetoric in Democracy: A Systemic Appreciation. *Political Theory, 38*(3): 319–339.

Hajer, M. A. (1995). *The politics of environmental discourse: Ecological modernization and the policy process.* Oxford: Clarendon Press.

Hawkins, K. W., & Linvill, D. L. (2010). Public health framing of news regarding childhood obesity in the United States. *Health Communication, 25*(8), 709–717.

Horin, A. (2008, November 22). Best defence in war on junk food ads is our island home. *The Sydney Morning Herald*. Retrieved January 16, 2013, from http://www.smh.com.au/news/opinion/adele-horin/best-defence-in-war-on-junk-food-ads-is-our-island-home/2008/11/21/1226770735299.html

House of Representatives (HoR) Standing Committee on Health and Ageing. (2008a, June 13). *Inquiry into obesity in Australia*. Adelaide: Hansard, Australian Government.

House of Representatives (HoR) Standing Committee on Health and Ageing. (2008c, September 11). *Inquiry into obesity in Australia*. Sydney: Hansard, Australian Government.

House of Representatives (HoR) Standing Committee on Health and Ageing. (2008g, November 26). *Inquiry into obesity in Australia*. Canberra: Hansard, Australian Government.

House of Representatives (HoR) Standing Committee on Health and Ageing. (2008i, December 8). *Inquiry into obesity in Australia*. Gold Coast: Hansard, Australian Government.

Johnson, G. (2010, October 28). Obesity is a big problem in need of big solutions. *The Sydney Morning Herald*.

Jones, M. D., & McBeth, M. K. (2007). A narrative policy framework: Clear enough to be wrong? *Policy Studies Journal, 38*(2), 329–353.

Kim, S.-H., & Anne Willis, L. (2007). Talking about obesity: News framing of who is responsible for causing and fixing the problem. *Journal of Health Communication, 12*(4), 359–376.

Lang, T., & Rayner, G. (2007). Overcoming policy cacophony on obesity: An ecological public health framework for policymakers. *Obesity Reviews, 8*(Suppl. 1), 165–181.

Lawrence, F. (2010, December 9). Extent of corporate influence on health policy revealed: Fast food and drink giants to help draft strategy. *The Guardian*. Retrieved January 17, 2013, from http://www.guardian.co.uk/politics/2010/dec/09/health-policy-extent-corporate-influence

Lawrence, R. G. (2004). Framing obesity. *The Harvard International Journal of Press/Politics, 9*(3), 56–75.

Lewis, S. (2011, April 3). Feeding frenzy. *The Sun Herald*. Retrieved January 17, 2013, from http://newsstore.fairfax.com.au/apps/viewDocument.ac;jsessioni d=A138BC13BDAECA126DCDC3931BDFD55E?sy=afr&pb=all_ffx&dt =selectRange&dr=1month&so=relevance&sf=text&sf=headline&rc=10&r m=200&sp=brs&cls=2924&clsPage=1&docID=SHD110403209IT2N3 06N

Maude, F. (2010, December 27). The nudge is no policy fudge. *The Guardian*. Retrieved January 17, 2013, from http://www.guardian.co.uk/commentisfree/2010/dec/27/nudge-fudge-community-level

Milne, S. (2010, November 17). The corporate grip on public life is a threat to democracy. *The Guardian*. Retrieved January 17, 2013, from http://www.guardian.co.uk/commentisfree/2010/nov/17/corporate-grip-public-private-sector

Pilkington, E. (2008, July 29). Eaten up. *The Guardian*. Retrieved January 17, 2013, from http://www.guardian.co.uk/environment/2008/jul/29/food.climatechange

Roe, E. (1994). *Narrative policy analysis: Theory and practice*. Durham, NC: Duke University Press.

Sheafer, T., Shenhav, S. R., & Goldstein, K. (2011). Voting for our story: A narrative model of electoral choice in multiparty systems. *Comparative Political Studies, 44*(3), 313–338.

Shenhav, S. R. (2005). Concise narratives: A structural analysis of political discourse. *Discourse Studies, 7*(3), 315–335.

Shenhav, S. R. (2006). Political narratives and political reality. *International Political Science Review, 27*, 245–262.

Shugart, H. A. (2011). Shifting the balance: The contemporary narrative of obesity. *Health Communication, 26*(1), 37–47.

Stark, J. (2008, August 21). Bloated obesity costs a threat to the nation. *The Age*. Retrieved January 17, 2013, from http://www.theage.com.au/national/bloated-obesity-costs-a-threat-to-the-nation-20080821-3zm2.html

Stark, J. (2011, January 16). Fast-food companies buying into healthier side. *The Age*. Retrieved January 17, 2013, from http://www.theage.com.au/national/fastfood-companies-buying-into-healthier-side-20110115-19s0y.html

Stone, D. A. (2002). *Policy paradox and political reason: The art of political decision making* (Rev. ed.). New York: W.W. Norton.

Swierstra, T. (2011). Behaviour, environment or body: Three discourses on obesity. In M. Korthals (Ed.), *Genomics, obesity and the struggle over responsibilities* (Vol. 18, pp. 27–38). London: Springer.

Szarka, J. (2004). Wind power, discourse coalitions and climate change: Breaking the stalemate? *European Environment, 14*(6), 317–330.

Thaler, R., & Sunstein, C. R. (2008). *Nudge: Improving decisions about health, wealth and happiness*. New Haven, CT: Yale University Press.

The Guardian. (2010, November 17). Letters: Food policy fears. *The Guardian*. Retrieved January 18, 2013, from http://www.guardian.co.uk/society/2010/nov/17/fast-food-policy-fears-bma

Van Hulst, M., & Yanow, D. (2014). From policy "frames" to "framing": Theorizing a more dynamic, political approach. *American Review of Public Administration.* doi:10.1177/0275074014533142.

White, M. (2010, December 1). Bufton Tufton spins in his grave. *The Guardian.*

Williams, R. (2011, February 27). Get set for our messiest food fight yet. *The Age.* Retrieved January 18, 2013 from http://www.smh.com.au/national/get-set-for-our-messiest-food-fight-yet-20110226-1b9b3.html

Wright, J. (2011, March 13). Obesity ads urge a swap for health. *The Sun Herald.* Retrieved January 18, 2013, from http://www.smh.com.au/national/obesity-ads-urge-a-swap-for-health-20110312-1bs1x.html

3

Defining the Scope of the Issue

Beneath the veneer of the simplistic environment-behaviour divide (recounted in more nuanced detail in the previous chapter), recent research has also begun to unpack the greater complexity and variety of constructions of obesity as a public problem. Though the temptation—certainly among proponents of the Structured Opportunity narrative—is to present the political debate as one between scientific experts and industry interests, what my analysis unveils is especially pointed disagreement *within* the expert community about the problem of obesity and its best solution. I will have much more to say about this in the coming chapters, but of particular focus here are the two emerging narratives that flank the dominant narrative and its primary counter, and which enjoy particular (and increasing) salience among recognised experts in this field. Indeed, central to their appeal is a sense that both the Facilitated Agency and Structured Opportunity accounts require too many 'leaps of faith' with respect to scientific knowledge on this issue—that the issue is unknowable in scientific terms with reliance just on the environmental (with respect to food and activity) and behavioural, in any mix; that no 'solution' associated with either of the dominant accounts is proven, or likely, to work. Instead, then, these two narratives shift the gaze away from the

J. Boswell, *The Real War on Obesity*,
DOI 10.1057/978-1-137-58252-2_3

environmental-behavioural and identify a different sort of problem at the source. They seek to reimagine the scope of the problem of obesity.

One greatly reduces the scope to the level of the individual, and the treatment, care, and attention that individuals dealing with obesity require. The obsession with population-level solutions, in this account, is speculative at best, and worse still ignores the plight of the millions already suffering due to obesity. So the focus comes on Individual Intervention. But, in line with the previous chapter's efforts to muddy the environmental-behavioural divide, this is not simply a manifestation of the hegemonic biomedical discourse in health. Individual Intervention can come in the form of an impersonal pill or procedure, but it can equally come in the form of counselling, comfort or, above all, caring.

The other narrative greatly increases the scope—obesity is, in this view, less a unique problem of an environmental, behavioural, or medical nature, and more simply one manifestation of a broader Social Dislocation. Yet, again, this is not simply the 'social determinants of health' in action. This account of Social Dislocation goes well beyond a concern for inequalities in health access and outcomes, and sees obesity itself as a pathology of a deeper socio-economic injustice.

The apparent goal is to challenge the focus of the 'main debate' discussed in the previous chapter and to promote a raft of alternative policy prescriptions for the problem of obesity. Certainly, battles over problem definition, and the scope that these definitions entail, have been a sustained focus of policy studies literature in relatively recent times precisely for this reason: setting the scope of the problem enables advocates of the status quo to restrict, and advocates of change to expand, the relevant range of stakeholders to involve and policy actions to pursue (see Jones and McBeth 2007). Yet in neither the Individual Intervention nor the Social Dislocation narratives does this entirely play out, or at least not as neatly as this policy studies maxim would allow. What my analysis shows is that the debate over scope is not purely a strategic function to further material interests or ideological commitments. Instead, I suggest that defining scope represents a crucial and further confounding aspect of the complex knowledge politics of obesity.

The structure of the chapter is as follows: I begin by outlining prevalent understandings about the scope of policy problems. I then recount the two expert narratives that flank the 'main debate', highlighting how they invert policy studies orthodoxy as it relates to the discursive battle over issue scope. I conclude by outlining the implications for how actors understand obesity in Australia and Britain and how they make and contest relevant knowledge claims through sites of democratic debate.

Defining Policy Problems: Contesting the Scope of Obesity

The battle over the scope of issues is a common point of interest in policy studies scholarship. It is best associated with the hugely influential Advocacy Coalition Framework, as one of the key components of political contestation. The simplified maxim is that those seeking to shore up the status quo try to restrict the scope of the issue, while those seeking to challenge it open up the scope to broaden horizons (see Sabatier and Jenkins-Smith 1999; Weible et al. 2011 for important reviews). Debating issue scope is regarded as a discursive strategy deployed by actors and is seen, in these stylised terms, as a key element of 'narrative policy tactics' by scholars who adopt a quantitative, positivist framework for understanding the impact of policy narratives (see Jones and McBeth 2007; Shanahan et al. 2011).

Yet, of course, the 'main debate' on obesity as described in the previous chapter does not seem to neatly fit this pattern. Both the Facilitated Agency and Structured Opportunity accounts present obesity similarly as representing a mix of environmental and behavioural factors. There is no effort by proponents of the Facilitated Agency narratives to deploy tactics to restrict the parameters of the issue—indeed, if this were the case, they would be fighting to make obesity an entirely private matter, which they avowedly are not.

Instead, my analysis in this chapter shows that debates over scope are not just a function of perceived interests, but are intimately related to competing claims to knowledge in this complex and uncertain area. The two expert-dominated narratives that I recount below challenge the assumptions about scope left unquestioned in the 'main debate'. Both are based on a scepticism—grounded, first and foremost, in the scientific evidence—about the prospect of achieving population-wide behavioural change, either through regulating the food environment or through nudging consumers (or in whatever mix of the two). The Individual Intervention account seeks to shrink the scope and bring to the fore knowledge about individual treatments. The Social Dislocation account seeks to expand the scope and bring forth knowledge about the broader implications of modernity and the prevalent socio-economic order. The former shrinks the scope in order not to reinforce the status quo but to buttress calls for new policies and much greater commitment of government resources; the latter expands the scope not to demand greater policy intervention but to, in many ways, underline the futility of any realistic policy action at all. Both accounts entail complex webs of relation with different sources of expert knowledge. I outline these complexities in detail in the accounts that follow. In doing so, what I hope to foreshadow, and will pick up again in much more depth in Part 2, is the impact both have on a festering expert dissensus on this issue.

Narrative 3: Individual Intervention

This narrative emphasises caring for and treating the millions of individuals who are already suffering or at risk of suffering the adverse health effects of obesity, as well as developing medical tools for preventing the condition in the first place. It is espoused most strongly by clinicians and allied health professionals, representatives of the pharmaceutical and medical equipment industries, and also by some patients and patient groups (Text Box 3.1).

The starting point of this narrative is not a generation or two ago, as with the pair of narratives in the previous chapter, but right back to the roots of human evolution:

Text Box 3.1

Individual Intervention

Essence
The obesity crisis has generated millions of victims who need immediate and ongoing medical help.

Main proponents
Clinicians, allied health professionals, pharmaceutical and medical equipment industries, patients

Characters
Villains: Food and weight loss industries
Victims: Those already obese
             Health service
Heroes: Health workforce

Targets of intervention
Treatments, hospitals, interdisciplinary clinics

Symbols and slogans
- The 'fragile' health service
- The 'super-obese'

Performance
- Authoritative
- Diffuse—sometimes shocking, rational, or empathetic

Eating is one of the strongest basic human instincts, stronger than sex. We have been genetically programmed to search for food from the time we were single-celled organisms swimming in the primordial swamp. But in the last 100 years, we have switched from food shortage to food abundance, and our bodies are still stacking up surplus spare energy in the form of belly fat and other spare tyres. (Proietto 2008)

The suggestion is that in order to survive people developed a powerful drive to eat, storing up on food when it was available in preparation for times of scarcity. As such, one affinity that it does have with the Structured Opportunity narrative in particular is that the big disruption has come through changes in the environment. The advent of modern society has transplanted people from a state of food scarcity to one of massive overabundance. Obesity is thus described in physiological terms as a 'normal response to an abnormal environment' (interview with a British clinician, May 2012).

According to the proponents of this narrative, industry is the chief villain, both the food industry and, especially for Australian adherents, the weight loss industry. Rather than providing a solution, these actors are seen as an essential part of the problem. They are seen as exploiting the growing market for dieting and weight loss products by selling people 'solutions' that are 'unsustainable' and more often than not actually contribute further to their obesity (interview with an Australian clinician, July 2011).

Government attempts to stem rapidly swelling rates of obesity through social awareness campaigns and community-based interventions are regarded as fruitless. Obesity, it is assumed, is a condition or even pathology that cannot be solved in the vast majority of cases simply by providing people with better information about nutrition and more opportunities to exercise, no matter how intensively the intervention is undertaken. Setting the scope at the level of the population is, in this sense, seen as pointless. A clinician explained:

> In the long term, if you follow any intense lifestyle program for obese people—whether you call it recidivism or recalcitrancy— [it will] fail. It is probably more to do with the unique physiology of being obese. Your physiology will drive you to eat back to the weight you were—unless you move to Ethiopia! (HoR Inquiry, May 12, 2008, p. 40)

This is not to say that some advocates of Individual Intervention do not also support calls for population-wide policy actions, in the form of taxes, subsidies, advertising restrictions, and so on. The point is that many still view these as hopeless both in preventing obesity and in helping those with the condition already. The support, in this sense, represents an expression of frustration at the problem and solidarity with others concerned, rather than any genuine belief in the prospect of impact. It is generally thought that efforts to impact on whole populations through public health measures are founded on ideology and hope rather than science. Most of these proposed regulations, it is thought, will make no difference but others might actually be counterproductive. For example, prominent British obesity physician and well-known advocate of the Individual Intervention narrative, Dr Ian Campbell (2011), argued against a 'fat tax' in a conservative British tabloid on the basis that it was impractical and unfair given the burden it would place on those of lower socio-economic status, echoing claims from food industry representatives that any such tax would be 'regressive' in nature.

Overall, it is felt that it is far more important to shrink the scope of the issue from the population level to the individual level. The chief way to approach this is by helping the growing numbers of people who are already obese. Indeed, obese individuals are seen as the forgotten victims, powerless to remedy the situation on their own in a spiral of ill-health and mental anguish.

The health service is equally represented as a victim, underfunded and ill-prepared to deal with the crisis. A rapidly growing number of 'super-obese' patients with multiple, complex chronic conditions is, according to some reports, already overwhelming the staffing and equipment capacity of hospitals. A report in the UK's *Daily Mail* tabloid suggested that 'some obese patients have been the victims of surgical errors and poor assessment of their needs, as well as a lack of staff and equipment to care for them safely' (Hope 2011). The primary care desperately needed to stem this flow is thought to be chronically underfunded, with general practitioners in both the UK and Australia actively discouraged by perverse incentive structures from helping patients manage their weight (interview with an Australian primary healthcare advocate, July 2011; interview with a British clinician, May 2012).

The heroic intervention in this narrative, then, is in the first place to pour resources into treating the victims of the obesity epidemic. Crucially, it is thought that this treatment should be provided by medical professionals in primary and acute settings across a variety of sub-disciplines—professionals trained to handle their patients safely and sensitively. One clinician explained at an HoR hearing:

> Health services are already busy looking after established old diseases and trying to deal with those issues, and they are finding it difficult to deal with obesity. So the first point we make there is the need for obesity to have a

coordinated model of care, particularly for child and adolescent service delivery, and the need to train health professionals in appropriate sensitive management of children and young people and their families. (HoR Inquiry, September 11, 2008c, p. 71)

The other key intervention is to boost investment into proven ways of helping those with or at risk of obesity. This is thought to include funding clinical research about promising pharmaceutical, surgical, and psychological treatments for the condition, as well as pouring resources into supporting primary care, providing additional staffing and equipment in hospitals, and initiating specialised training of medical professionals. A doctor specialising in primary care for obesity explained in a column for the *Sunday Age*:

The facts are that lifestyle change is hard—it is complex, time-consuming and requires a long-term view, often stretching to years. Families have to be ready for and helped with change. Funding and resources for crucial well-trained nurses and allied health professionals (dietitians, psychologists, physical activity experts) is sparse within our current health-care system. [But] we know that the only proven, effective way to treat children with obesity is through intensive treatment by a range of health professionals. (McCallum 2008)

Performing the Individual Intervention Narrative

The Individual Intervention narrative is performed by a diverse cast, with support from clinicians, like bariatric surgeons, general practitioners, psychologists, and dietitians, as well as medical researchers, equipment providers, and some patient groups and individual patients. Though there is little specialisation in relation to which sites the actors perform in—with many spanning both public and elite sites—there is a notable difference in terms of how different types of actors do so. Some proponents convey a sense of urgency about the need for investment in medical interventions by attempting to shock. They recall exotic anecdotes about grossly obese patients or present striking images about the medical complications associated with obesity. For example, witnesses from KCI Medical Australia, an equipment supplier, enacted Individual Intervention by confronting committee members at one HoR hearing with graphic photos of obese patients suffering with chronic wounds (HoR Inquiry, September 11, 2008c, p. 9)—an occasion which one committee member recalled as being particularly gruesome and affecting (interview with a member of HoR Committee, May 2011).

Some practitioners, on the other hand, seek to convey a calm assuredness through a very measured and gentle tone, reinforcing their message that obese individuals can be saved through the assistance of qualified professionals like them. A particularly common refrain in interviews was for actors to bemoan the 'schizophrenic' coverage of obesity in the media—one minute a crisis needing urgent attention, the next a light-hearted matter of retrograde 'fat-shaming' in shows like *The Biggest Loser*. Many spoke of their desire to present a much more sensible and positive message publicly. Likewise, a well-known Australian weight management physician told me that he consciously removed 'the "O" word' from his vocabulary because he saw how much damage that label could do to the self-esteem of his patients, thereby worsening their plight considerably (interview with an Australian clinician, June 2011).

Other adherents to this narrative perform it in a way that is emotional and involving. They convey empathy for the suffering of obese individuals, through harrowing anecdotes about personal struggle or loss of dignity. For example, one Australian clinician articulated the Individual Intervention narrative at an HoR hearing as follows:

One of my colleagues in South Australia who runs the obesity services in Royal Adelaide Hospital was discussing with me just last week a patient, a 270-kilogram young woman, whom the ambulance officers could not get from her home to outpatients. Eventually she went by truck. There were issues in actually getting her to outpatients. In the end the consultation was conducted in the car park, which is a highly unsatisfactory forum in which to have your consultation and there is no possibility of physical examination. (HoR Inquiry, May 12, 2008, p. 33)

Narrative 4: Social Dislocation

This narrative is salient in the UK—particularly within the left-wing press—but is only engaged with on the very margins of the debate in Australia.[1] It holds that rising rates of obesity are indicative of a deeper societal malaise; they are thought to be just one manifestation (among many) of the profound inequality and social dislocation that the modern economic and political systems generate. The scope here, then, is widened from beyond the individual and their interaction with the environment (in terms of food and physical activity) to encompass the entire socio-economic foundations of contemporary liberal democracies like Australia and Britain (Text Box 3.2).

For proponents of the Social Dislocation account, the problem is best symbolised by evidence about the socio-economic gradient on obesity, whereby those with low education and income are far more likely to be obese and suffer the associated health complications. As *Guardian* columnist Polly Toynbee (2007) argued:

> Fat is a class issue. Obesity is mainly a disorder of the less well off, an added stigma to a life of low esteem, making a poor life worse.

Unlike the narratives discussed so far, the starting point in this narrative is not a nostalgic look back at better times. Instead it is a sense that good food, nutrition, and health have always been class-related. According to this narrative, the particular set of circumstances that have led to increasing rates of obesity (as opposed to underweight and malnutrition) involve not so much rising rates of poverty but rising rates of social inequity, and changes in how such socio-economic disadvantage is manifested:

---

[1] Though some actors in Australia adhere to it privately, they do not perform it publicly, or at least not in the context of political debate. This is, in broad terms, consistent with what Olsen et al. (2009) find in their assessment of submissions to the HoR Inquiry. I will discuss this phenomenon of self-censorship in much more detail in Chap. 8, but at this point it is important to foreshadow that this discrepancy between the cases is instructive about the relative performance of the UK debate, and the way in which advocates pursue their cause therein.

Text Box 3.2

Social Dislocation

Essence
The obesity crisis is a manifestation of deeper social problems due to inequality.

Main proponents
Public health academics, left-wing commentators

Characters and causation
Villains: Neoliberalism and its proponents
Victims: The underclass
Heroes: Defenders of equality

Targets of Intervention
Inequality and the policies and practices that reproduce it

Symbols and slogans
- The socio-economic gradient
- 'Fat is a class issue.'
- 'Future?...What fucking future?'

Performance
- Moral and intellectual righteousness
- Air of futility

No longer fighting communicable diseases like their Victorian predecessors, public health specialists are faced with social and lifestyle issues such as obesity, smoking, drug misuse, teenage pregnancy and stress-related disorders .... While the challenges have changed, the inequalities remain, and many practitioners argue that the underlying barrier to improving public health is still poverty ... and the gap is widening. (Hempel 2008)

Yet, importantly, this is about more than the 'social determinants of health'. At root the conceptualisation of the problem (and ramifications for its solution) is much deeper. The neoliberal economic order is held to be responsible for the development of a highly sophisticated but ultimately amoral system of food production, which creates incentives for the promotion of profitable but unhealthy items at the expense of more nutritious ones. As one *Guardian* journalist explained: 'communities around the planet have been disempowered by a system that appears to offer an abundance of cheap food, but in reality dictates unhealthy and limited choices to an overworked and underpaid workforce that cannot afford any better' (Pilkington 2008). It is this 'broken' system, therefore, that ensures that junk food is often very cheap and supplied in larger, more calorific quantities in developed countries like Britain.

Just as significantly, neoliberal policies—which have been so aggressively promoted across so many areas—are considered key contributors to the demoralisation of large swathes of society, leaving them more vulnerable to the seduction of unhealthy food products. The working class and especially underclass are depicted as victims, with their agency severely limited by the sense of depression and dislocation the wider economic system engenders, manifested primarily in desperate, antisocial behaviours like drinking, smoking, and overeating. This point is poignantly illustrated in a *Daily Mail* article about the relationship between health and life prospects in a derelict industrial town in South Wales. In it a local man (reported to be 'clutching a can of lager in the street') told an interviewer: 'It doesn't bother me that I may not get to 70 or even 60 .... Future, what fucking future?' (*Daily Mail* 2011).

Health promotion efforts are thought to have failed partly because they harass individuals who are poorly educated and incapable of processing the information and taking the opportunities that are presented. More importantly, though, these activities are also seen as chastising and further alienating individuals who already feel economically marginalised and socially isolated. Sir Michael Marmot (2010), perhaps the most eminent public health expert in the UK and certainly the best known advocate of this narrative, argued in a column in the *Guardian*:

> Put simply, childhood deprivation, the stress of poverty, overcrowding, living in a run-down area, feeling powerless at work and being unemployed do not give people the control over their lives that fosters good health and enables them to succeed in making difficult changes in behaviour.

The crusading efforts of public health campaigners, too, are seen by many proponents of this narrative as incapable of making a big difference (though many still support these moves in some form). Big Food is represented as little more than a symbol of the prime culprits, which are the broader political and economic systems that produce and sustain such companies. The problem, for them, is not *McDonald's* but the system which supports and maintains *McDonald's*. As such, proponents of this narrative see that vilifying that company (or any other equivalent) actually means missing the more significant point. For example, a *Guardian* columnist explained of the push for whole-of-population policies on nutritional labelling and advertising of junk food:

> Would that make much difference? Every little helps, as they say. But frankly, the task is gargantuan. (Toynbee 2007)

For proponents of this narrative, the inevitable result has been unprecedented increases in rates of obesity. But they contend that the big problem is that this increase, and associated burden on the health system, is by no means the only crisis facing government. They suggest that other 'wicked' problems like climate change, crime, and social exclusion are at least equally pressing, and they are seen as equally rooted in systemised greed, individualism, and inequality. The belief is that obesity is simply a symptom of an unjust and unsustainable approach to organising society. As such, current attempts to deal with these issues are thought to be indicative of an antiquated model of public service that is ill-equipped to cope with the complex, multifaceted problems wrought by the neoliberal context in which it operates:

> Another day, another headline: today obesity, tomorrow teenage pregnancy, the day after crime figures. Social problems operate a revolving-door policy these days. As soon as one goes away, another turns up. For the most part, these problems are regarded as entirely separate from each other. Obesity is a health issue, crime a policing issue and so on. So the government launches new initiatives here, there and everywhere, builds new hospitals, puts more money into the police and prisons. And there's little real hope of improvement. (Crace 2009)

The heroic intervention involves a need for 'integrated thinking', at the heart of which is a fairer approach to income distribution (interview with a British public health researcher, January 2012). This single action, it is thought, would turn around rates of obesity, as well as cure any number of other social ills. Marmot again put it this way:

> The health and wellbeing of today's children and of those children when they become adults depends on us having the courage and imagination to do things differently, to put sustainability and wellbeing before a narrow focus on economic growth and bring about a more equal and fair society. (Quoted in the *Daily Mail* 2010)

However, the majority of proponents of this narrative are not hopeful that any such move will be forthcoming in the foreseeable future, given the considerable 'political obstacles' in the way (interview with a British public health researcher, April 2012). For them, obesity and all the other social ills caused by the neoliberal order are therefore likely to persist and should be mitigated in the most enlightened and humane ways—hence adherents of this narrative typically promote the targeting of resources and support to poor neighbourhoods and at-risk ethnic minorities.

Performing the Social Dislocation Narrative

The Social Dislocation narrative is voiced publicly by a narrow band of proponents in the UK (though, to reiterate, it is almost completely absent from public debate in Australia), with adherents among academics and left-leaning media commentators. These proponents typically adopt a sense of righteousness. This is both moral, in that they present themselves as the true defenders of the underclass, and intellectual, in that they present themselves as being the only participants in the debate able to make the analytical leap from thinking of obesity as a health issue to thinking of it as a social one. One striking example was at an open board meeting of the FSA, on June 11, 2008, when Professor Sue Atkinson, a strong proponent of the Social Dislocation account and long-time member of the board, made a point of challenging the presentation of a bureaucrat from the Department of Health about the government's proposed obesity strategy. In line with the Social Dislocation narrative, she pointed to problems associated with rapidly rising costs of food and growing social inequities. The bureaucrat (who performed the Facilitated Agency narrative) responded with a long-winded explanation about the changing landscape of food consumption in Britain and the move towards healthier products. Atkinson waited for him to finish before authoritatively offering her interpretation of the data—that it was overwhelmingly wealthy people moving towards these products rather than the 'at-risk' groups she expressed concern about. She was courteous and rational, as befitted the norms of the site, but nevertheless conveyed a sense of superiority. Her performance showed that she was, as an independent public health expert, able to see the true nature of the problem (both normatively and empirically) in a way that he and his colleagues either could or would not.

In the media, in line with the sense of futility with which this narrative concludes, this righteousness is often augmented by an air of anger and despondency at the status quo. This is encapsulated in one journalist's review of Jamie Oliver's *Ministry of Food* series:

> Miss this *Ministry of Food* series and you'll be missing some of the most powerful political documentary in years. In it, whether by intention or accident, the naked chef has entered the domestic life of a British town and captured a snapshot of the country's social health. The result is an indictment of the current political system as disturbing as any ideological tract. Food, and real people's experience of it, is still all about class. (Lawrence 2008)

Managing the Scope of Obesity

To reiterate, the orthodox understanding in the policy studies literature is that competition over the perceived scope of a public problem represents an effort to control policymaking resources. In broad terms, the understanding is that those preoccupied with maintaining the status quo seek to restrict the scope of problem definition, while those advocating for change seek to expand it. Here, however, we see that these dynamics can in fact be much more complicated.

In the first account discussed above, the efforts of Individual Intervention proponents to narrow the scope of obesity are not about maintaining the status quo as such. They are better understood as being about underpinning a claim for greater resources and attention for the neglected and under strain provision of adequate health services. This appears to be a significant challenge to the status quo imbued by the dominant Facilitated Agency narrative. Yet embedded in this very challenge is a return to an older orthodoxy. The individual qua patient may be the key motivating appeal of this narrative, but the Individual Intervention narrative makes them a subsidiary of policy action. Narrowing the scope makes the targets of intervention, in a policy sense, much more familiar and tractable agents: clinics, health professionals, carers. Policymakers know how to deal with these targets. They know how to identify them, manage them, measure their performance, and so on. In pragmatic policymaking terms, then, the Individual Intervention account has distinct appeal over the woolly, amorphous, and/or difficult targets of the dominant pair of narratives discussed in the previous chapter. Importantly, too, we should not even understand claims for greater resources as being about buttressing the status quo in health services provision. Accounts of Individual Intervention can seamlessly encompass both the narrow biomedical understanding and the broader emerging holistic approach to preventing, treating, and caring for obesity at the individual level. It is only very occasionally presented by proponents of the Individual Intervention narrative as being one at the expense of the other.

On the one hand, then, the Individual Intervention narrative entails an epistemic repudiation of the New Public Health. On the other hand, though, it does not necessarily entail a return to the biomedical paradigm, making space as it does for myriad emerging forms of medical evidence and experiential practitioner expertise. This dual dynamic is indicative of the complex, porous, shifting relationships in the knowledge politics of obesity. I will return to these tensions and overlaps in greater detail in Chaps. 5 and 7 when I seek to unpack consensus and dissensus about expert knowledge.

Returning to the point about scope first, though, in the second account we should equally see the Social Dislocation account in a different light to what is suggested by the dominant Advocacy Coalition Framework

(ACF) understanding of this dynamic. The efforts of proponents of the Social Dislocation narrative to broaden the scope of the problem cannot be neatly understood as merely seeking to underpin change.

Of course, at one level, that seems the obvious goal of their advocacy. By linking obesity to much broader social and economic forces, the proponents of Social Dislocation seek to challenge the validity of prevailing policies (such as social marketing). But, at another, the Social Dislocation narrative speaks to a broader, deeper sense of futility about any action at all. Unlike the other three narratives discussed so far, Social Dislocation is perhaps more properly understood as critique rather than a complete narrative. A critique, for Roe (1994), is a cogent challenge to dominant interpretations but one which fails, on its own terms, to make sense of a clear alternative course of action. In this sense, the Social Dislocation account of obesity is pitted against the dominant (and key counter) understandings of the issue. However, the very broad scope that this challenge engenders means that the prescriptions suggested in its denouement do not, or at least are not intended by its proponents to, represent a pragmatic course of action. The target—the neoliberal social and economic order—is simply too big. It is in this sense the very opposite of Individual Intervention. For the most part, too, proponents of the Social Dislocation narrative seem all too aware of the futility of their interpretation—such that, as I will dwell on in Chaps. 8 and 9, many are unwilling to voice this narrative publicly at all for fear of being seen as irrelevant/impractical (most acutely, of course, in the Australian case where this narrative is almost completely latent).

The effect, returning to the ACF account of competition over scope, is that proponents of Social Dislocation actually serve to undermine apparent allies within the same broad 'public health' coalition. Their half-hearted support for regulatory reforms is undercut by a broader narrative that trivialises the importance of these manoeuvres. All that is left is the reluctant concession that 'every little helps'. And so the move to broaden the scope of the issue does little to promote genuine change, but plenty to complicate the contest over knowledge and meaning in this public health crisis.

Conclusion

This discussion here has paved the way for my analysis of the factions and alliances, overlaps and discrepancies that characterise the knowledge politics of obesity in Australia and the UK. By outlining the two narratives that flank the 'main debate' about agency on this issue, I have illustrated how expert advocates of these accounts have attempted to reimagine the scope of obesity, and thus shift the gaze of policymakers, in diametrically different directions. The Individual Intervention narrative narrows down the scope, and in the process targets the proposed reforms at the familiar institutions, actors, and practices of healthcare policy. The Social Dislocation account greatly broadens the scope, targeting instead (at least rhetorically) the very economic and social foundations of the modern democratic state. The presence of these flanking, expert-led narratives has important implications for what and whose knowledge is deemed to count with respect to this issue, who gets to represent that knowledge credibly in debate, and how it filters through eventually to policymaking. I will deal with these intricate complexities in the advocacy of obesity experts in subsequent chapters through Part 2 of this book.

What I turn my attention to next, though, are the remaining two narratives uncovered in my analysis. These are two contrasting accounts that equally remain largely marginalised, but by no means ignored, by recognised obesity experts in Australia and Britain. Yet their marginalisation does not make them unimportant—in fact, I will suggest that their relative silence in elite deliberations actually speaks volumes. I argue that for quite different reasons their positions on the margins of debate make them especially important for understanding both the complex contest over knowledge and meaning on this issue, and the implications this has for policymaking in both countries.

References

Campbell, I. (2011, October 4). UK obesity experts debate if Danish fat tax is right for Britain. *The Mirror*. Retrieved January 15, 2013, from http://www.mirror.co.uk/news/technology-science/uk-obesity-experts-debate-if-danish-83163

Crace, J. (2009, March 12). The theory of everything. *The Guardian*. Retrieved January 15, 2013, from http://www.guardian.co.uk/society/2009/mar/12/equality-british-society

Daily Mail 2011, 'Future? What "f****** future?" The British estate where "healthy" life expectancy is just 58.8 years', The Daily Mail, February 12. Retrieved January 17, 2013, from http://www.dailymail.co.uk/news/article-1356247/Gurnos-Merthyr-Tydfil-The-British-estate-healthy-life-expectancy-just-58-8-years.html

Hempel, S. (2008, November 19). Why poverty remains the greatest barrier to change. *The Guardian*.

Hope, J. (2011, July 27). Parents "are just ignoring child obesity warnings". *The Daily Mail*. Retrieved January 16, 2013, from http://www.dailymail.co.uk/news/article-2019166/Child-obesity-Parents-ignore-warnings-heavy-handed-tactics-waste-time.html

House of Representatives (HoR) Standing Committee on Health and Ageing. (2008c, September 11). *Inquiry into obesity in Australia*. Sydney: Hansard, Australian Government.

House of Representatives (HoR) Standing Committee on Health and Ageing. (2008d, September 12). *Inquiry into obesity in Australia*. Newcastle: Hansard, Australian Government.

Jones, M. D., & McBeth, M. K. (2007). A narrative policy framework: Clear enough to be wrong? *Policy Studies Journal, 38*(2), 329–353.

Lawrence, F. (2008, October 1). Britain on a plate. *The Guardian*. Retrieved January 17, 2013, from http://www.guardian.co.uk/lifeandstyle/2008/oct/01/foodanddrink.oliver

Marmot, M. G. (2010, August 15). Ignorance is as big a killer as obesity. *The Observer*. Retrieved January 17, 2013, from http://www.guardian.co.uk/commentisfree/2010/aug/15/michael-marmot-health-wellbeing

McCallum, Z. (2008, April 27). Far too much to lose. *The Sunday Age*. Retrieved January 17, 2013, from http://www.theage.com.au/news/opinion/far-too-much-to-lose/2008/04/26/1208743319461.html

Olsen, A., Dixon, J., Banwell, C., & Baker, P. (2009). Weighing it up: The missing social inequalities dimension in Australian obesity policy discourse. *Health Promotion Journal of Australia, 20*(3), 167–171.

Pilkington, E. (2008, July 29). Eaten up. *The Guardian*. Retrieved January 17, 2013, from http://www.guardian.co.uk/environment/2008/jul/29/food.climatechange

Proietto, J. (2008, February 19). Surgery will do more than education to fix the obesity epidemic. *The Age*. Retrieved January 27, 2013, from http://www.theage.com.au/news/opinion/surgery-will-do-more-than-education-to-fix-the-obesity-epidemic/2008/02/18/1203190737640.html

Roe, E. (1994). *Narrative policy analysis: Theory and practice.* Durham, NC: Duke University Press.

Sabatier, P., & Jenkins-Smith, H. (1999). The advocacy coalition framework: An assessment. In P. Sabatier (Ed.), *Theories of the policy process* (pp. 117–166). Boulder, CO: Westview Press.

Shanahan, E. A., McBeth, M. K., & Hathaway, P. E. (2011). Narrative policy framework: The influence of media policy narratives on public opinion. *Policy & Politics, 39*(3), 373–400.

The Daily Mail. (2010, February 14). Plans to raise retirement to 68 will fail because three-quarters of us will be too ill to work. *The Daily Mail.* Retrieved January 17, 2013, from http://www.dailymail.co.uk/news/article-1250129/ The-rich-live-seven-years-longer-poor-people.html

Toynbee, P. (2007, October 19). We need to start a social revolution by truly putting children first. *The Guardian.* Retrieved January 18, 2013, from http://www.guardian.co.uk/commentisfree/2007/oct/19/comment.children

Weible, C. M., Sabatier, P. A., Jenkins-Smith, H. C., Nohrstedt, D., Henry, A. D., & deLeon, P. (2011). A quarter century of the advocacy coalition framework: An introduction to the special issue. *Policy Studies Journal, 39*(3), 349–360.

4

Disputing the Problem

Where the previous two chapters focused on the key contending narratives in elite deliberation on obesity—the main debate over agency and the more niche expert debate over the scope of the issue—this final chapter in Part 1 focuses on two narratives at the margins of elite debate. One is a Nanny State narrative, whose proponents blame rising rates of obesity on obese individuals themselves and the experts and policymakers who apologise for and enable their behaviour. The other is a Moral Panic narrative, whose proponents see concerns about obesity as a 'beat-up' that further, and unnecessarily, stigmatises obese individuals.

At first glance, these two narratives may seem to have little in common. The Nanny State account is associated with a reactionary or 'toxic' interpretation that actively vilifies obese people; the Moral Panic account is associated with a sociological perspective that evinces a strong empathy for obese people. The former is enacted in a detached, matter-of-fact tone; the latter typically contains weighty emotional content. The former is typically associated with right-wing chauvinism; the latter with left-wing feminism. Indeed, these are accounts that at their core seem to be underpinned by very different views of human nature and different visions of the good society. Yet despite these discrepancies, there are also

© The Editor(s) (if applicable) and The Author(s) 2016
J. Boswell, *The Real War on Obesity*,
DOI 10.1057/978-1-137-58252-2_4

some surprising commonalities between these two accounts that render their side-by-side comparison here fruitful.

First and foremost, these are narratives that bring overriding assumptions about the need for any 'war on obesity' into question. They deconstruct, in order to dispute, the very existence of the supposed policy problem. Proponents of the Nanny State narrative are deeply critical of the construction of obesity as a public concern. To them, this is not an issue that the state should be involved in at all. They wish instead to return obesity to the realm of the private. And proponents of the Moral Panic account want something similar, and for only slightly different reasons. Instead of disputing the 'publicness' of obesity, they dispute its problematisation. They question the strength of the science linking obesity to ill-health and paint the 'war on obesity' as the highest profile and perhaps most damaging venture in ill-informed 'fat discrimination'. And so, like proponents of the Nanny State narrative, they see obesity as properly kept in the realm of the private.

Second, what follows from this questioning of the problem itself is that in practice both are pushed to the margins of political debate on obesity. Proponents of each are opposed to the 'public health' orthodoxy and the elite expert knowledge that typically informs debate and policymaking on this issue. This is not to say they do not possess expertise themselves, nor that they do not draw on the same sorts of evidence that other actors in debate do—a point I will stress and draw out in the following chapters. Yet in setting themselves up against the dominant orthodoxy pervading the other four narratives discussed thus far—the shared premise that rising rates of obesity are a significant public problem in need of policy attention—both are greeted with hostility by other actors. The Nanny State account is actively seen as dangerous and excluded from elite debate, more so in Australia where it has become completely taboo. The Moral Panic narrative is seen as more well-meaning but as equally misguided and dangerous, and is, as I shall show, consciously squeezed into the margins of both debates, again more clearly and acutely in the Australian case.

Exploring these two narratives adds considerable nuance to existing scholarship on the social construction of obesity. Analysing the Nanny State account not only helps to go further beyond the parsimonious individual/behavioural categorisation apparent in older studies to unveil deeper complexities, but also challenges widespread assumptions—

especially within the public health scholarly community—about the supposed pre-eminence of the Nanny State image in political debate (see Swinburn 2008). I show that far from dominating discussion, the Nanny State narrative is actually more of a ghost stalking elite debate from the margins (for more on this, see Boswell 2015). Analysing the Moral Panic account, on the other hand, presents a newly emergent construction of obesity which itself has origins in social science scholarship of this phenomenon. So, where the Nanny State narrative is more marginal than existing scholarship seems to hold, the Moral Panic narrative is actually, in contrast, more embedded in political debate than the prevailing Fat Studies scholarship would suggest.

But exploring them also speaks to broader work in policy and politics on marginal policy actors and their efforts to impact the public agenda. The bulk of this literature focuses on strategies that might enable such groups to get their issues on the agenda, as well as on how powerful elites seek to thwart their efforts. Here, in contrast, we see actors who would like to have obesity *removed* from this agenda. The effect of their efforts on public discourse has implications for broader work on agenda-setting, opening up important new avenues of research inquiry.

In this chapter, I start by briefly laying out the policy studies literature on marginal interests and agenda-setting. I then set the contrasting narratives side by side, presenting both narratives before comparing their similarities—in content and in effect—in the penultimate section. This enables discussion of the broader implications for the relevant policy studies literature. The broader aim though, in the context of the book, is to lay the groundwork for the subsequent analysis in Part 2, where I delve deeper into the implications of the contending narratives on obesity for policy work in this field.

Defining Policy Problems: Contesting the Agenda

No aspect of policymaking has animated as much interest in recent decades as agenda-setting (see Baumgartner and Jones 2009; John et al. 2013; Dowding et al. 2010). The primary focus, herein, is on the inputs to the policymaking process, in terms of the demands made by citizens and lobbyists, and their impact on the agenda for legislative attention. Indeed, such is the focus on this element of the policy process that in many respects agenda-setting, and its link (or lack thereof) to public opinion, has come to completely dominate discussion about the quality of democratic policymaking in different political contexts (see Sabl 2015).

One of the hopes that I have for the analysis in this book is that it will temper this emphasis and begin the task of casting much brighter light on the important democratic deficits that occur through the policy process, as public debate feeds into elite deliberations and, ultimately, policy action (see Boswell forthcoming for much more on this). Indeed, in my conclusion I will call for more attention, among analysts, policymakers, and civil society actors, 'downstream' in the policy process. But, before getting there, in this chapter I want to stress that my analysis confounds, and therefore contains important lessons for, mainstream scholarship on agenda-setting, too.

Specifically, the orthodox assumption in the agenda-setting literature is that vulnerable or marginalised actors compete to get attention. And the relevant literature focuses largely not only on the extent to which they are successful in different contexts (see Baumgartner and Jones 2009), but also on the obstacles to and enablers of such success, and the strategies and practices adopted therein (see Kingdon 1995). Much is known about the struggle of such groups to promote their issues onto the public agenda. Agenda management, or issue neutralisation, in contrast, is typically presented as a strategy or practice of powerful elites who would deny actors such voice (Gustafsson and Richardson 1979; Thacher and Rein 2004). Echoing (and of course in many ways related to) the orthodox claims in policy studies about issue scope in the previous chapter, the primary emphasis in this literature is on how powerful actors (industry lobbyists and political elites) work to maintain the restrictive status quo and prevent the broadening out of policy attention.

Yet the pair of narratives I identify in this chapter invert this relationship. With respect to obesity in Australia and the UK, marginal actors want this issue *off* the agenda. They do so for different reasons—advocates of Nanny State narrative do not see obesity as a *public* problem;

advocates of the Moral Panic account do not see it as a *problem* at all— but both equally present a challenge to the expert and elite consensus about the need for government action on this issue (albeit a consensus fractured among the narratives described in the previous two chapters). These actors are not, of course, able to manage the issue off the agenda. In fact, as I will show, as a consequence of their combative challenge they are largely excluded from elite and expert sites of deliberation and decision-making. But as I foreshadow here, and will go on to explore in much greater detail in Part 2, they play a crucial role in the broader dynamics of agenda management and issue neutralisation which see the war on obesity at risk of petering out. Their challenge to the very presence of a public problem conditions the way that proponents of other narratives perform their accounts, further confuses and confounds the knowledge politics of obesity, and brings the legitimacy of policymaking of the issue into question. I outline the contrasting narratives now before returning to this issue in the discussion towards the end of the chapter.

Narrative 5: Nanny State

Some actors in both Australia and the UK put the blame for obesity on the shoulders of the 'nanny state'. The essence of this narrative is that rising obesity is due to state interference and a decline in personal responsibility. Adherents to this narrative therefore regard growing rates of obesity as a direct consequence of interventionist policies. Their catchcry is to ask: 'Where is the call for personal responsibility?' (C Akroyd in the *Sun Herald* 2008) (Text Box 4.1).

In Australia, this narrative builds on key strains of national identity, particularly the image of Australians as robust and self-sufficient. Its starting point is decades ago, when Australians were thought to have taken responsibility for their own health and well-being, based on the assumption that discipline and personal accountability are qualities that abounded in the past. As one proponent of this narrative explained in his correspondence to a conservative tabloid:

> **Text Box 4.1**
>
> **Nanny State**
>
> *Essence*
>
> Rising obesity is due to excessive government interference in the health service.
>
> *Main proponents*
>
> Libertarian and conservative commentators and think tanks
>
> *Characters*
>
> **Villains:** Government, Obese people, Health do-gooders
> **Victims:**   Taxpayers
> **Heroes:**   Free marketeers
>
> *Symbols and slogans*
>
> - 'Nanny State'
> - 'Where's the personal responsibility?'
>
> *Performance*
>
> - Acerbic
> - Aggressive
> - Concerted

I grew up in the '40s and '50s and lived in a housing commission home. My mother worked full-time and my stepfather was away working five days a week. There was no obesity, we walked to school or rode our bikes. Fast food consisted of Weet-Bix for breakfast. (C Akroyd in the *Sun Herald* 2008)

In the UK, proponents of the Nanny State narrative pin the rise in obesity to declining moral fibre—a common trope among conservative commentators on political and social issues in that country (Edgar 2008). It is thought that rising obesity reflects a society that fosters the wrong sorts of qualities. A columnist for a conservative broadsheet surmised:

[The idea that] our obesity epidemic is the fault of junk-food outlets and confectionery suppliers … is a mindset that is fostered by cynical politicians who see few votes in telling people that which discomforts them, even if it's the truth. Much better to identify a 'dark force' and then roll out an initiative to tackle it. This exculpates the guilty, while creating an impression of activity. (Randall 2009)

In both cases, it is the intervention of government that is seen to have disrupted the happy equilibrium afforded by a culture of personal responsibility. The key villain in this narrative, the state itself, is regarded as having indulged in an ill-advised and ultimately doomed attempt to assert control over the population and 'save people from themselves' (Barnes 2009). The problem, as it is perceived, is that government has been too willing to pick up the tab for obese individuals' chronic ill-health. This is seen to have sent out the wrong sort of message to individuals in the community. A commentator in the *Age* put it this way:

These days most people understand the risks of drugs, tobacco, alcohol and bad nutrition and the benefits of moderation, if not abstinence. But if people choose freely to take health-threatening risks ... perhaps they should not assume that the community will always cheerfully clean up after them. (Barnes 2009)

Recent, misguided government attempts to address the issue are seen to have been aided by health professionals and academics. Whether out of ambition or ideology, these experts are seen as encouraging state overreach. A UK columnist in the *Telegraph* said:

I was surprised to see a top medic describe morbid obesity as a 'disease' on the BBC News. Surely this insults patients who have no control over their maladies. (Pelling 2007)

Indeed, for proponents of this narrative, campaigns and interventions are not just futile but counterproductive, compounding the problem by reducing individuals' sense of personal responsibility. The result, it is thought, is that the other key actors in this debate, obese people themselves (and parents of obese children), have taken advantage of this state of affairs. As such, the constant intervention of the lecturing 'Nanny

State' is assumed to be a causal factor in the rise of obesity. An editorial in a conservative Australian broadsheet concluded:

> Resisting temptation is one of life's lessons. By asking for a tougher regulation, parents are asking the state to let them off the hook. (*The Australian* 2008)

According to proponents of this narrative, skyrocketing treatment costs have put enormous pressure on inefficient health services, with the potential to bankrupt the government in the process. Jeremy Sammut (2008, p. 37) of conservative Australian think tank the Centre for Independent Studies (CIS) concluded in his submission to the HoR Inquiry:

> Unless we look beyond the false promise of more spending on prevention, and start to address how to move beyond relying on taxpayers to finance the accelerating cost of health care into the twenty-first century, Medicare is going to impose unsustainable burdens on future generations.

The heroic intervention depicted in this account is for a shift away from the 'safety blanket' model of health provision. The targets of intervention include the cast of villains outlined earlier—both obese actors themselves and the policymakers and professionals who excuse and enable their behaviour. As such, this intervention entails that policymakers should stop enabling the destructive lifestyle of obese individuals by treating them as victims. Instead, it is thought that people must be encouraged or even forced to take responsibility for themselves. One correspondent to a progressive British broadsheet voiced this opinion bluntly:

> I say take away free healthcare. If you had to fork out for every trip to the NHS, you would be less inclined to over-indulge. ('Ravenlighte' in the *Guardian* 2008)

Chris Berg (2008) of the conservative Australian think tank the Institute of Public Affairs proposed the same solution more eloquently in his newspaper column:

The only way to avoid [an ever-expanding health budget] is to drop the conceit that all medical problems are public problems, and to reintroduce the idea that individuals should be responsible for their own health.

Performing the Nanny State Narrative

The Nanny State narrative finds voice through a narrow band of actors, largely opinion writers and lay correspondents in newspapers in both countries. These actors typically make a point of being plain speaking and using common sense. They enact this narrative by adopting an aggressive and acerbic tone that reinforces their scepticism about government and expert interference. One colourful example appeared in an opinion column for an Australian tabloid:

> Among the most irritating requests for government overreach arising from the Rudd Government's 2020 summit was the proposal that we all do government-approved exercise every day. I first suspected this was designed by an infiltrating cell of small-government activists to deliberately ring the emergency George Orwell-alarm, but no such luck. Po-faced do-gooders actually canvassed the idea that we should perform state-approved calisthenics. (Wilkinson 2009)

This is even the case with the more dignified performances of this narrative. Elite actors tend to convey the same sense of cynicism and appeal to common sense found in the media opinion columns. For instance, in the UK, Conservative MP Phil Davies asked incredulously in response to his own party's obesity policy announcement: 'Why are we so wedded to the nanny state?' (quoted in White 2010). Likewise, in his submission to the HoR Inquiry the CIS's Jeremy Sammut (2008) expressed contempt for public health experts and their push for greater emphasis on prevention and primary care:

> the merry-go-round continues. Governments readily look to spend even more on prevention policies that have not improved the overall health of the population, and which have actually presided over the emergence of the so-called obesity 'epidemic.'

Narrative 6: Moral Panic

This narrative sees growing concern about an 'obesity epidemic' as sensa-tionalist, opportunistic, and ultimately damaging. It is on the margins of the various sites of debate across both countries, promoted mainly by a minority of academics,[1] a handful of media commentators and some com-munity activists. These proponents do not deny that obesity has increased in prevalence in the community, but they believe that the extent of this increase and the strength of its links to ill-health have been massively over-stated. They argue that the hysteria over obesity is just a form of discrimina-tion, as Donna Simpson, a community activist and subject of a story in the *Guardian*, concluded: 'I think people worry about health because it's the easiest place to hang fat hatred' (quoted in Cowell 2010) (Text Box 4.2).

This narrative does not begin with a nostalgic vision of fit and lean individuals, however. Instead, it adopts a historical perspective that peo-ple have always come in all shapes and sizes—that obesity is not a new phenomenon, and that body image has long been an issue of scrutiny and discrimination (see Gard and Wright 2001; Lupton 2013). What is thought to have changed, and worsened, the situation is the rising rheto-ric around the 'obesity epidemic'. Obesity, in this sense, is seen to have been constructed as grotesque, undesirable, and extremely dangerous to one's health. A journalist for the *Sunday Age* opened her story with the following passage on childhood obesity:

> It used to be dismissed as puppy fat. A chubby child who looked like a mini Michelin Man was once considered cute, their excess weight a passing phase that posed no cause for alarm. That was before childhood obesity was declared a 'national emergency'. Before parents were warned that excess skin folds and a craving for cupcakes could consign their child to an early grave. (Stark 2009)

For proponents of the Moral Panic narrative, researchers, clinicians, and, more sinisterly, medical industry and pharmaceutical representa-tives are the villains responsible for this state of affairs. They are seen to

---

[1] There is in fact a small body of interdisciplinary scholarship under the umbrella of 'fat studies' that plays a crucial role in underpinning this narrative. See Solovay et al. (2009). Lupton (2013) pro-vides a compelling account of a similar perspective in brief form.

Text Box 4.2

Moral Panic

Essence

Obesity has been unreasonably constructed as a crisis by vested interests.

Main proponents

Academics, media commentators, community activists

Characters

Villains: Big Pharma and the 'medical industry'
Victims: Obese people
Heroes: Activists

Targets of intervenon

The ill-conceived 'war on obesity'

Symbols and slogans

- 'The obesity myth'
- 'Health At Every Size'

Performance

- Diffuse—sometimes calm and rational, indignant, satirical

have misled policymakers about the prevalence of obesity and its associated ill-effects for personal gain. Australian journalist Richard Guilliatt (2009) explains that new evidence which throws doubt on claims of an obesity epidemic has met with hostile reaction from the 'scores of medical researchers, diet companies, gastric banding surgery entrepreneurs and drug companies whose interests are tied up with the obesity debate'.

To compound matters, many of the public policies and medical practices deployed and promoted in the name of the 'obesity epidemic' are seen as discriminatory. It is felt that the majority of medical practitioners in particular adopt a moralising attitude towards their patients that is alienating. Australian academic Jenny O'Dea, who is an outspoken advocate of the Moral Panic narrative, explained in a sound bite for the *Sunday Age*:

there's going to be a backlash from parents who are offended and affronted when they have a big child and the dietitian or the doctor or the teacher assumes that they've been neglecting that child .... They assume that this mother mustn't know about fruits and vegetables, that they allow their child to sit in front of the TV all day eating chips and soft drink. In reality the child has always been big since birth, the family are big and the child is healthy and growing beautifully and should not be stigmatised by uninformed health professionals who just make an instant assumption. (J. O'Dea, quoted in Stark 2009)

Under this narrative, current policies designed to address the 'obesity epidemic' are regarded not just as prejudiced but as entirely counterproductive. They are thought to have actually worsened the problem of unhealthy lifestyles, making food and activity matters of 'anxiety or obsession' rather than fun (interview with an Australian nutrition researcher, June 2011). If anything, it is thought, this has trapped many obese individuals in a cycle of mental anguish which results in less exercise and worse nutrition. What is more, adherents to this account believe that far more serious problems may have emerged, with a spike in the numbers of people who suffer from eating disorders and malnutrition resulting from attention to the so-called 'obesity epidemic'. A prominent Australian academic and her colleagues conveyed this point sombrely in their submission to the HoR Inquiry:

We argue that the very public attention on fatness as abhorrent promotes self-monitoring and weight management practices that are dangerous for children and young people. While some of this becomes evident in the prevalence of young people with eating disorders, we would also argue from our research that a preoccupation with being thin or not being fat is very common among young people. Food and activity become associated with the amount of 'energy in and out'. This approach, common in the cultures within schools and in school curricula and teaching about health, leaves out the pleasures of moving competently, and the complexities of our relationships with food. (Wright et al. 2008)

The end result, it is thought, is that obese individuals have become victims of demonisation. The moralising of public health experts, politicians, bureaucrats, and others in society is seen to reinforce long-standing discriminatory practices against those who fail to conform to body image norms. One member of the public suggested in a letter to the editor of an Australian tabloid:

> This constant finger wagging and bullying is creating unwarranted and unhealthy pressures on people. The once natural act of energy consumption has become so infused with mainly negative emotions and obsessional thinking of feared consequences that eating habits have been elevated to an expression of a person's integrity and morality. (S. Romei in the *Daily Telegraph* 2008)

The heroic intervention in this narrative is for a calmer, more rational approach to the issue. The targets of intervention, in this sense, are the actors who problematise obesity, not those who are obese or who cause obesity. These are the researchers who myopically exaggerate the dangers of the so-called 'fat bomb'; the clinicians who bluntly target and stigmatise the obese individuals in their care; and, most of all, the ignorant policymakers who pursue the foolish 'war on obesity'. In concrete terms, then, this intervention means toning down the emphasis on obesity altogether, and instead promoting practical strategies for helping the vulnerable and embedding healthy lifestyles in a positive way. For instance, in her appearance as a witness at an HoR hearing, O'Dea explained to the committee the potential for 'getting more bang for your buck socially and physically' from incorporating a range of positive, fun, and culturally appropriate messages around nutrition and activity (HoR, Sydney hearing 2008, pp. 45–46).

In the UK, there has been particular emphasis on the concept of Health At Every Size (HAES). This involves encouraging everyone to get fit and active rather than worry about their weight. One expert explained the necessary intervention in an opinion column for the *Guardian*:

> The demand for weight-loss pills and surgeries, fuelled by the notion that everyone has a moral obligation to achieve a slim body, will continue to eat up more and more of increasingly precious NHS budgets. This is what awaits us (or worse), if we don't change direction and stop trying to follow the one-size-must-fit-all method of healthcare. Health researchers and professionals who have become disenchanted with the failure—and dangers—of a traditional weight-centred approach to health are increasingly adopting

the Health At Every Size philosophy ... HAES emphasises the benefits of sound nutrition, active living and body confidence as ends in themselves, not as a route to weight management. (Aphramor 2009)

Performing the Moral Panic Narrative

The Moral Panic narrative is performed by a cast of different actors, incorporating public health and sociological researchers as well as journalists and commentators all of quite different political persuasions—libertarian, feminist, and social constructivist. These actors generally perform in distinct, specialised settings—the journalists narrating in the media and the researchers narrating in more elite sites. They also narrate in quite different ways. The performance of a public health expert at a hearing of the HoR Inquiry, for instance, drew heavily on the logic of the scientific method and her *ethos* as an objective and rational voice in an otherwise commercialised and politicised debate. The centrepiece around which her testimony was based was a simple graph mapping some of her research. This served as a prop both to clearly communicate her message and to impress on them the scientific rigour of her approach (interview with an Australian nutrition researcher, June 2011). In contrast, the most prominent performance of this narrative in the Australian press drew much more heavily on the emotions. In a magazine-style article dominated by photos of an idyllic backyard setting, the author presented the struggle of the parents of a 'cherubic' young girl branded by experts as obese (Guilliatt 2009).

But, in its exclusion from most expert and elite deliberations, the Moral Panic account has also been performed satirically with an intention to provoke a response. A good example can be found in an article in the *Guardian* that highlighted the activism of 'gainers' who deliberately gain weight in defiance of conventional public health expertise and societal norms (Cowell 2010). There was doubtless an element of voyeurism and novelty that attracted the attention in the first place. For these activists, it is their very embodiment of the obesity (see more in Chap. 5), and pointed inversion of the shame typically associated with it, that strengthens their message. In Australia, a handful of media reports reproduced similar themes. Particularly striking was a report that enacted the Moral Panic narrative through shocking humour, encapsulated in the large and striking inset image of the 'Aqua Porko' synchronised swimming team in action (Lentini 2011).

Conditioning the Agenda: The Mainstream Impact of Marginal Narratives

The at times acerbic or satirical tinge to both these contrasting narratives is indicative of their shared fate in political debate. Pushed to the margins, distrusted, and deemed dangerous by the majority of recognised policymaking elites and experts in Australia and the UK, the response of proponents of both is to undermine and lampoon these establishment figures, and their assumptions about an 'obesity epidemic'. This shared fate is instructive about the broader political debates on obesity and foreshadows much of the discussion that will occupy Part 2 of this book.

For one thing, it tells us not so much about what type of knowledge matters for policymaking on this issue, but about how the representation of that knowledge matters: how its performance, and its performers, condition its influence on policy discussion and decision-making in this contested area. As I shall explain, actors engaged in these debates have been keen to reflect on the importance of the 'packaging' of knowledge claims on obesity in policy debate. In the case of both these narratives, the 'packaging' is what engenders marginalisation. Despite protestations to the contrary from proponents—indeed, as I will show in the following chapters, both are avowedly 'evidence-based' accounts according to many of their advocates—both are perceived to be grounded stridently in alternative forms of knowledge to the prevailing preference for EBPM. The Nanny State narrative, for instance, is associated with a form of cultural knowledge or assumed common sense that is pitted against 'the evidence'; it is seen to embody the damaging stereotypes that public health advocates must fight against. The Moral Panic narrative, too, is perceived as being based in idiosyncratic forms of personal experience that fail either to grasp important epidemiological principles (primarily that what holds for individuals has little bearing at the population level) or to hold up against professional expertise ('They should come and see my clinic', one British clinician suggested dismissively). Either way, the explicit message is that these are not credentialed experts and, with an obvious ideological or personal axe to grind, they should not be taken seriously in debate.

But at the same time, the implicit message is that both actually are taken seriously in debate. Their relative absence from elite deliberations, in this sense, speaks volumes. The obvious concern is that both fundamentally call into question the meaning and purpose of the 'war on obesity', however that might be understood or conceived.

The trouble with the Moral Panic narrative specifically is that it introduces further doubt to the knowledge politics of obesity. Proponents in Australia and Britain are cast as 'obesity deniers' with other actors making frequent analogies to climate change scepticism. Yet such an analogy can only stretch so far, because the degree of expert 'consensus' around obesity remains fragile, if not entirely fractured. Many of the criticisms and concerns advanced by proponents of the Moral Panic account in scientific terms—about the effects of social marketing, about the impact of tax increases or labelling regimes, about the science surrounding surgical and pharmaceutical interventions—overlap precisely with the claims made by proponents of the other narratives, echoing the broader dissensus surrounding this issue.

Moreover, the Moral Panic narrative is not, as with climate change scepticism, for example, entirely without expert backing. In fact, it has close affinities with a rich vein of scholarship in the social sciences about stigmatisation, public health, and weight (best encapsulated in the interdisciplinary subfield of 'Fat Studies'). And it enjoys support from a small but vocal handful of clinical and epidemiological researchers (underpinning the Health at Every Size movement). So, as a credible threat to the very existence of obesity as a public problem, the Moral Panic narrative adds significantly to the doubt, and thus conflict, surrounding the expert politics of this issue. This is something I explore in much more detail in Chap. 7.

The Nanny State account presents a quite different challenge. The worry is that this narrative is potentially dominant, not marginal; that it appeals to the narrow prejudices of the broader public, and thus threatens to undermine the prospect of reasoned policymaking on this issue. This is the view that the majority of actors I spoke with subscribed to. As such, my noting of the absence (in Australia) or lack of prominence (in the UK) of the Nanny State narrative from elite deliberations represented, for them, a welcome finding.

Yet, to be clear, these two fates (absence and lack of prominence) are not identical, and here the comparison between cases becomes useful. On the few occasions when elite actors, or actors in elite venues, voiced the Nanny State narrative about obesity in the UK, this was clearly not the case. Indeed, their claims prompted a great deal of interest and debate, with elite actors gaining much publicity in their rebuttal of the Nanny State account. Professor Steve Olds' opinion piece in the *Guardian*, for example, which gave voice to at least some important elements of the Nanny State narrative, prompted public health experts and community activists to restate and reimagine their refutation of the populist claims he invoked. Lord Lawson's Nanny State claims on obesity in the House of Lords, too, provoked an outpouring from the community of actors committed to government action (of various kinds) on obesity, justifying their positions in ways that more closely engage with the populist resistance. Conversely, it has been the taboo surrounding the Nanny State narrative in Australia that serves to stunt and 'close down' debate in that country. On the one hand, it denies representation to a popularly held narrative, in the process fuelling resentment and a sense that democratic policymaking occurs primarily by stealth. On the other hand, the taboo barring the Nanny State narrative in Australia can also condition and cow the advocacy of the very actors who seek to limit its spread. In the UK, where elite expressions of the Nanny State narrative have occurred from time to time (and been engaged with vocally by other actors), this narrative is considered a constituent but minor view within the broader debate. But in Australia, where the Nanny State narrative has become completely taboo and has not been engaged with, there is an acute sense of looming threat among elite actors about the prevalence of this perspective in the broader public sphere. Where none of my UK interview participants mentioned the term 'Nanny State' unless prompted by my questioning, many of their counterparts in Australia volunteered it early and often in interviews. One interview participant even began our interview by almost instantly claiming:

The term they use in the debate is the 'Nanny State'. It's very, very effective. So as soon as it's not personal responsibility … when we demand action, they always fall back on the Nanny State". (Interview with the Australian public health advocate, April 2011)

Moreover, the same participants also reflected that their public statements were conditioned by fear of being cast as a proponent of the Nanny State (the image itself, not the narrative that lampoons it), leading them to mute or muffle some of the bolder ideas they believed in. Indeed, there is a notable link here to the point raised in the previous chapter: that though the Social Dislocation narrative has enjoyed traction both in the public sphere and in some elite sites in Britain, it has been almost completely absent from the Australian debate (supported in Olsen et al. 2009). Despite the fact some interview participants reported to me in private that they saw considerable value in the Social Dislocation narrative none were willing to advocate it publicly for fear of a backlash. The sense overall, then, is that the 'ghost' of the Nanny State stalks elite deliberations in Australia. The conscious exclusion of this narrative weakens perceptions of legitimacy among populist critics and, just as importantly, among the other political actors themselves—a point I return to in Part 2 and the concluding discussion, where I flesh out the implications of this important discrepancy between the two cases.

Conclusion

For now, though, I return to the key takeaway messages from the analysis in this chapter. The first is that, in line with the work done in the previous two chapters in Part 1, my analysis here confounds typical assumptions in the literature on the social construction of obesity. Rather than centring around a debate over agency versus structure, or around the appropriate scope of the issue at hand, these two narratives actually challenge assumptions about the presence of a significant public problem with respect to obesity. The Nanny State narrative questions the publicness of the problem, while the Moral Panic narrative questions whether it is really a problem at all. Combined with the insights from the previous two chapters, we are beginning to see a much more complex, nuanced set of contending and overlapping interpretations about the nature of obesity than that typically revealed in the broader literature on this topic.

The second is that these findings have great salience for policy and politics scholarship on the battle over the public agenda. The radical narratives here work to get obesity *off*, not *on*, the public agenda. This challenges the prevailing orthodoxy in the agenda-setting literature and opens up new possibilities or avenues for inquiry in this subfield. Certainly, these are dynamics that seem to be equally at play in other contested areas such as climate change, indigenous rights or social exclusion (see Boswell 2015). The negating or challenging of the public agenda from the margins deserves more sustained attention in this subfield.

But I want to end Part 1 by discussing how these key insights build towards the analysis in Part 2. What I have shown here is that although the performance of these radical narratives does not serve to manage the agenda, it can be seen to play indirectly into the neutralisation of the issue. I reveal that the Moral Panic account, though it remains on the fringes of the debate, plays an important role in exerting influence from the margins. Its very denial of the problem further confounds and confuses the far-from-settled science of obesity, unsettling the prospects of even thin scientific consensus on this issue. It provides more ammunition for powerful 'merchants of doubt' (Oreskes and Conway 2010) to neutralise any sense of political urgency and dampen the appeal of radical policy action. I show that the Nanny State account is not a dominant rendering of the behavioural discourse, but a fringe—indeed, in Australia, taboo—narrative that shapes or conditions debate from the margins. Its position in debate speaks to broader concerns or dilemmas about the elite or expert-dominated nature of the political debate on this issue. It raises questions about the legitimacy that a debate of such character can (or, more pertinently, cannot) bestow on the policy work that follows—representing the key emphases of Chaps. 5 and 6. Likewise, the Moral Panic account thus brings into focus twin features of the knowledge politics of obesity—dissensus over the meaning of relevant scientific evidence, and uncertainty over the implications for policy making—that will be the broader focus of Chaps. 7 and 8, respectively. I turn my attention to this range of broader implications now as I move into Part 2 of the book.

References

Aphramor, L. (2009, May 9). All shapes and sizes. *The Guardian*. Retrieved January 15, 2013, from http://www.guardian.co.uk/commentisfree/2009/may/09/obesity-weight-health

Barnes, T. (2009, September 29). Good health, a responsibility not just a right. *The Age*. Retrieved January 15, 2013, from http://www.theage.com.au/opinion/society-and-culture/good-health-a-responsibility-not-just-a-right-20090928-g95q.html

Baumgartner, F., & Jones, B. (2009). *Agendas and instability in American government* (2nd ed.). Chicago: University of Chicago.

Berg, C. (2008, January 6). Tackling obesity – Should the public pay?: The case against. *Sunday Age*. Retrieved January 15, 2013, from http://www.ipa.org.au/news/1523/tackling-obesity---should-the-public-pay-/category/9

Boswell, J. (2015). Toxic narratives and the deliberative system: How the ghost of nanny stalks the obesity debate. *Policy Studies, 36*(3), 314–328.

Cowell, L. (2010, March 18). The women who want to be obese. *The Guardian*. Retrieved January 15, 2013, from http://www.guardian.co.uk/lifeandstyle/2010/mar/18/women-obese-donna-simpson-gainers

Dowding, K., Hindmoor, A., Iles, R., & John, P. (2010). Policy agendas in Australian politics: The governor-general's speeches, 1945–2008. Australian *Journal of Political Science, 45*(4), 533–557.

Edgar, D. (2008, September 26). If Britain is a broken society, it's the Tories what broke it. *The Guardian*. Retrieved January 15, 2013, from http://www.guardian.co.uk/commentisfree/2008/sep/26/conservatives.britishidentity

Gard, M., & Wright, J. (2001). *The obesity epidemic: Science, morality and ideology*. New York: Routledge.

Guilliatt, R. (2009, May 8). Off the scale. *The Australian*. Retrieved January 16, 2013, from http://www.theaustralian.com.au/news/features/off-the-scale/story-e6frg8h6-1225710631861

Gustafsson, G., & Richardson, J. J. (1979). Concepts of rationality and the policy process. *European Journal of Political Research, 7*(4), 415–436.

House of Representatives (HoR) Standing Committee on Health and Ageing. (2008, September 11). *Inquiry into obesity in Australia*. Sydney: Hansard, Australian Government.

John, P., Bertelli, A., Jennings, W., & Bevan, S. (2013). *Policy agendas in British politics*. Basingstoke: Palgrave Macmillan.

Kingdon, J. W. (1995). *Agendas, alternatives and public policies*. London: Longman.

Lentini, R. (2011, April 8). Why should bigger women apologise? *The Daily Telegraph*. Retrieved January 17, 2013, from http://www.dailytelegraph.com.au/news/opinion/why-should-bigger-women-apologise/story-e6frezz0-1226035562526

Lupton, D. (2013). *Fat*. London: Routledge.

Olsen, A., Dixon, J., Banwell, C., & Baker, P. (2009). Weighing it up: The missing social inequalities dimension in Australian obesity policy discourse. *Health Promotion Journal of Australia, 20*(3), 167–171.

Oreskes, N., & Conway, E. M. (2010). *Merchants of doubt*. New York: Bloomsbury Press.

Pelling, R. (2007, October 17). State schools are to blame, not Oxbridge. *The Daily Telegraph*. Retrieved January 17, 2013, from http://www.telegraph.co.uk/comment/3643394/State-schools-are-to-blame-not-Oxbridge.html

Randall, J. (2009, February 5). We're in denial: Afraid to face up to the real causes of recession. *The Daily Telegraph*. Retrieved January 17, 2013, from http://www.telegraph.co.uk/finance/comment/jeffrandall/4528718/Were-in-denial-afraid-to-face-up-to-the-real-causes-of-recession.html

Sabl, A. (2015). The two cultures of democratic theory. *Perspectives on Politics, 13*(2), 345–365.

Sammut, J. (2008, April 33). Healthy lifestyles are taxing for everyone. *The Australian*.

Solovay, S., Wann, M., & Rothblum, E. (Eds.). (2009). *The fat studies reader*. New York: NYU Press.

Stark, J. (2009, August 5). The fats of life: When chubby's no longer cute. *The Sunday Age*. Retrieved January 17, 2013, from http://www.smh.com.au/lifestyle/diet-and-fitness/the-fats-of-life-when-chubbys-no-longer-cute-20090905-fc5b.html

Swinburn, B. A. (2008). Obesity prevention: The role of policies, laws and regulations. *Australia and New Zealand Health Policy, 5*, 1–7.

Thacher, D. & Rein, M. (2004). 'Managing value conflict in public policy'. *Governance, 17*, 457–486.

The Australian. (2008, May 19). More nanny state. *The Australian*. Retrieved January 17, 2013, from http://www.theaustralian.com.au/news/more-nanny-state/story-e6frg72o-1111116374935

The Daily Telegraph. (2008, June 21). Your say … *The Daily Telegraph*.

The Guardian. (2008, April 23). Joe Public views from Society's blog: Is the nanny state becoming too bossy? *The Guardian*.

The Sun Herald. (2008, October 26). Letters to the editor. *The Sun Herald*.

White, M. (2010, December 1). Bufton Tufton spins in his grave. *The Guardian*.

Wilkinson, C. (2009, December 2). Politicians should stop banning our fun. *The Sydney Morning Herald*. Retrieved January 18, 2013, from http://www. smh.com.au/opinion/society-and-culture/politicians-should-stop-banning-our-fun-20091130-k0zl.html

Wright, J., Gard, M., Tinning, R., Cliff, K., Garrett, R., O'Flynn, G., et al. (2008). *Submission to the house of representatives inquiry into obesity in Australia*, no. 19 (Inquiry into Obesity). Australian Government, House of Representatives, Canberra.

Part II

Policy Engagement

5

Representing Knowledge

I saw the scales tip at [an obese weight]. I realised that I really had a problem, and that how could I as someone who is a representative of a group of people talk about the need for healthy lifestyles and the need for sensible eating when I was grossly overweight? People expect some form of hypocrisy from their politicians but certainly I would have no credibility in prosecuting that case if I wasn't actually practising what I preach. (Interview with an Australian politician, May 2011)

Though delivered in a light-hearted fashion, the quote above, drawn from an interview with one of the committee members involved in the Weighing it Up Inquiry, is indicative of something important about the representation of knowledge claims about obesity across both cases: that the public most affected by this issue, obese people themselves, do not have a strong or recognised voice. Indeed, if the universal fetish for evidence was what struck me most about the debate as I began my fieldwork (see the next chapter), what sunk in later as the most profoundly noteworthy feature of these debates was the fact that almost none of the actors actively engaged in Australia or Britain are themselves obese. This is not to say that there are no obese people among the elite of policymaking in both countries. There remain, of course, some obese politicians and

© The Editor(s) (if applicable) and The Author(s) 2016
J. Boswell, *The Real War on Obesity*,
DOI 10.1057/978-1-137-58252-2_5

policymakers that observers of politics in both countries could point to. What matters is that, like the committee member suggests above, these individuals are not deemed to have credibility in discussing a policy problem that they themselves embody.

I do not point this out in order to reductively condemn all other elites in this debate as callously reproducing 'fat hatred'. They are not consciously ignoring the claims of obese individuals and targeting them as a problematic group to be excluded and marginalised. On the contrary, most of these actors present themselves as actively and empathetically *representing the obese*. While a minority of actors who support the Nanny State narrative have been openly hostile or scornful towards obese people, the vast bulk of actors engaged in debate—those who subscribe to every other narrative—actually express deeply sympathetic views about the health problems and social discrimination that obese people disproportionately confront. They have, as I have shown, variously sought to advocate policy changes to eliminate, lessen, or remedy these problems on behalf of the obese people affected. The common refrain to evidence, which I will stress in the subsequent chapter, is a crucial element of this empathy—it is by reference to the facts in their entirety, rather than prejudicial assumption alone, that all these advocates represent obesity as much more than a personal failing. Their expertise on the matter allows them to represent the affected individuals so long at the centre of social scorn. The obese may not speak, but they are very much spoken for.

In this chapter, I look across the key narratives on obesity identified in Part 1 and identify the manner in which proponents of each attempt to represent the obese people at the centre of this policy debate. The findings uncover three sets of expert representative claims or identities, dubbed Role Model, Carer, and Nanny. Each is (outside proponents of the acerbic Nanny State account, at least) seen to be motivated by empathy towards those affected by obesity, but at the same time to have the effect of diminishing the perceived agency and capability of obese individuals, and omitting the crucial affective or emotional side to this issue. Ultimately, I argue that the absence of obese voices from the debate is a significant problem which limits and distorts democratic policymaking on obesity, in a way that directly undermines the (generally) good intentions of the advocates involved, regardless of their preferred narrative on the issue.

This chapter proceeds in three parts. In the first, I draw together evolving ideas about representation in democratic governance with recent work on the social construction of obesity. In the second, I present the analysis of the three primary representative claims or identities mobilised by actors in this debate, illustrating how they align with and cut across the narratives identified in Part 1 of the book. In the third, I conclude by considering the implications of these representative claims for obese people and their role in the political debate on this issue.

Speaking for the Obese: Networked Governance, Representation, and Policy 'Targets'

The notion of representation has long been central to the function of democratic governance. Stylised notions of a principal–agent relationship between representatives and their constituents—more often than not simplified down to the level of electoral mandate—have, in recent times, had to confront the complex subtleties of the differentiated polity (see Saward 2009). Networked governance has become the norm (with respect to obesity as much as any other issue). All sorts of actors exercise more or less legitimate claims to representation, and those claims can be as much based on knowledge as they are on office. Indeed, the surfeit of task forces and other such innovations to guide obesity policymaking in both countries, few of which have had their legitimacy questioned, and certainly never so for lacking a mandate, is testament to this.

In the midst of this shift in orthodoxy has been a swelling interest in representation of the affected citizens at the centre of public policies. There is a widespread push to better involve citizens more in the governance of complex and contested issues. Yet of course there are significant obstacles to achieving this in practice—the whole affected public cannot be consulted. It needs representatives. And how those representatives are identified and chosen remains a matter of ongoing contention.

Broadly speaking, there are two competing orientations to how this might be achieved in a context of networked governance: descriptive representation, or discursive representation. The former, associated with work on gender and ethnic minority representation, asserts that representatives should themselves emanate from the affected public and represent their descriptive features (Phillips 1995; Mansbridge 1999). The latter asserts that what matters is not descriptive features of individual representatives but that they are able to give voice to one of the key discourses (or, in the language of this book, narratives) that shapes political debate (Dryzek and Niemeyer 2008). The perceived advantage of discursive representation over descriptive representation is that it enables representation of affected interests that cannot represent themselves (its proponents largely have in mind future generations, animals, and so on).

Yet this distinction is also useful in thinking about representation of problematic 'target' groups in fields of social policy. In practice, many affected interests continue to occupy the role of passive objects of policy intervention. Smokers, substance abusers, the homeless, the unemployed, recidivist criminals, and so on have historically been unlikely to play an active part in the process that leads to relevant policies. Indeed, those who embody the deviant condition or characteristic under discussion are implicitly, or even explicitly, seen to make 'bad representatives' in empirical terms (they cannot represent themselves adequately) and normative terms (they ought not to be granted representative status). As such, their representation is typically discursive rather than descriptive. They retain a stigma which means that their representation typically comes through competent and empathetic outsiders rather than from actors who themselves embody the particular deviant characteristic.

Of course, as was made clear in the introduction, obesity has also long been imbued with just such a social stigma, at least in the Anglo sphere and Western Europe. Obesity is treated as a by-product of individual indulgence in the 'deadly sins' of sloth and gluttony (Dixon and Broom 2007). And so in this sense it is not entirely surprising that the obesity debates in Britain and Australia are so markedly dominated by the thin and fit. But what does this prevalence of discursive, rather than descriptive, representation imply for the affected interests at the centre of this issue?

As I have discussed at length already, the initial (and, for a few authors, enduring) reaction to the arrival of obesity on the public agenda in such circumstances was to perceive an extension and acceleration of 'fat hatred' or 'fat blaming'; rather than just being seen to hurt themselves, obese individuals are increasingly seen to also cause wider damage through their lack of self-control. Moreover, the creeping 'responsibilisation' of public health is thought to have further marginalised the obese as immoral, weak, and incapable (LeBesco 2011; Saguy 2013). In the morality tale laid bare by critical analysts, obese people are treated as *villains*, presented (unfairly) as deserving of public scorn and ridicule. Indeed, at its most extreme, the argument here is that the obese are portrayed as 'domestic terrorists' through the 'micro-fascist' practices of public health elites (see Rail et al. 2010).

However, as I have tried to argue in this book so far, such an account represents just one narrative of obesity (the Moral Panic account) among the many that contest the meaning and nature of this issue. In fact, as I showed in the last chapter, there is a swelling tide of experts and activists who draw on expertise to claim that obesity is caused by a range of socio-economic, environmental, genetic, psychological, and cultural factors. Explicit 'fat hatred' has become almost taboo, such that the Nanny State narrative that best approximates this view is not even represented in elite or empowered policymaking settings in Australia—a point I touched on in the previous chapter and will return to in Chap. 8. The key point to bear in mind here, though, is that for the most part obese people are represented as *victims* in both countries, deserving of support and encouragement.

This is not to cast the critical account about the obesity debate aside. Indeed, as the quote which began this chapter would suggest, a status of victimhood retains remnants of the older, stigmatising morality tale. And while explicit expressions of 'fat hatred' may have waned from elite discourse, obese individuals, and their personal experiences of obesity, remain excluded from key settings of political debate on this important public policy issue. So this raises the question of how these more sympathetic accounts of obesity as a public problem—how these discursive representatives—present knowledge claims on behalf of the obese individuals at the centre of this issue; how, and to what effect, do elite actors claim to represent the obese?

The analysis in subsequent sections outlines three core representative claims that align, or cut across, the competing narratives on obesity. They are represented for clarity in the box below and then fleshed out in detail in the discussion that follows (Table 5.1).

Table 5.1 How actors claim to speak for the obese

Narrative	Representative	Claim	Basis
Facilitated Agency People have forgotten how to lead healthy lifestyles due to big social changes, so they now need help relearning the basics.	Political or community/ cultural leader	Role Model— either actors who have 'been there, done that' or else elites who consciously model healthy behaviour	Action/ Experience
Moral Panic Obesity has been unreasonably constructed as a crisis by vested interests.			
Individual Intervention The obesity crisis has generated millions of victims who need immediate and ongoing medical help.	Professional/ Practitioner	Carer	Proximity
Structured Opportunity The obesity crisis is a direct consequence of industry excess and a lack of regulation.			
Social Dislocation The obesity crisis is a manifestation of deeper social problems due to inequality.	Scientific expert	Nanny	Distance

The Role Model

One key representative claim centres around the elite advocate as Role Model. The image underlying this account sees obese people *currently* as victims of circumstance, albeit as *potentially* active agents in their own cause. The obese are, in this account, unrealised heroes in their own personal redemption tale. The Role Model is, given these affinities, tightly associated with the Facilitated Agency narrative.

For proponents of this account, the Role Model's task is to help individuals realise the agency they possess in order to take control of their own weight and health. Crucially, this is to be achieved by example rather than through persuasion: Role Models represent obese people as much by their deeds as by their words. This is the claim underlying much of the funded government activity on obesity prevention in both Australia and the UK—in the social marketing campaigns, exercise and kitchen-garden interventions in schools, and so on.

But more commonly the Role Model is embodied in high-profile individuals. Celebrity chef Jamie Oliver has long occupied this role in Britain, such that he remains a 'go-to' authority in the media for response to government initiatives and controversies associated with obesity, and a common point of reference in debate.[1] The key figure of reference in Australia has been Tony Abbott, previously Minister of Health (then later Leader of the Opposition and Prime Minister). Abbott's well-known commitment to an active, healthy lifestyle represented model behaviour that citizens ought to follow.

Of greater interest still are the most compelling Role Models in the political discussion—those whose authority is based on their past experience. These elites are ideal Role Models because they used to be obese themselves. Indeed, it was the desire to be a Role Model that prompted the Committee for the HoR Inquiry, referenced in the opening vignette

---

[1] It is interesting to note—in line with the observations in the next chapter about the complexities of the competing narratives over time and across venue—that Oliver is not exclusively associated with the Facilitated Agency narrative, and at times reproduces (or is identified as reproducing) the Structured Opportunity narrative. Indeed, at the time of writing, he is a key campaigner in the push for a sugar tax in Britain. More often, however, he occupies the position a Role Model who exemplifies and seeks to inspire the lifestyle change perceived as necessary to combat obesity.

of this chapter, to embark collectively on a weight-loss regimen. Chair Steve Georganas explained at the outset of a hearing halfway through the Inquiry:

> We have taken an initiative, as a committee, this week. We have a booklet where we are monitoring what we are eating, what we are doing and what exercise we are doing. Most of us, I think, committed to starting off with this committee and doing something. (HoR Inquiry, June 20, 2008, p. 1)

Nevertheless, consistent with the shifting scope of obesity from private to public, the majority of Role Models line up behind the Facilitated Agency account and evince a sense of deep sympathy for obese people. Indeed, central to their claim is a shared experience with obese people that unites them against the thin, holier-than-thou 'zealots' who otherwise dominate debate. One Australian politician explained:

> I am interested with this term 'junk food'. I never agreed with it. I think it's a term that becomes purely pejorative. The food that goes in it seems to be subjective as to what someone's view is of junk food. Certainly sugar, salt, fat all those things—but what's junk and what is a genuine treat, you know, that kind of thing is not clearly defined. Once again that goes back to the zealots of the world. The zealots say it's all bad. And you yearn to try and find them eating doughnuts. And sometimes you do! (Interview with an Australian politician, June 2011)

As well as the understanding that comes from shared experience, Role Models also offer hope. This was most frequently apparent in the testimony of witnesses to the Parliamentary Inquiries in Australia. Weight Watchers Australia even recruited two of its clients—one being the 'Slimmer of the Year' for 2008—to tell their personal 'success stories' in their allotted time at one of the Weighing it Up Inquiry's public hearings. Indeed, reflecting on the broader experience of the Inquiry, one of the MPs on the committee referenced in the opening vignette was explicit about the perceived Role Model role:

> So, it's certainly given me a personal focus and whenever I can, when I'm speaking to the wider community—mostly I do that through regular

interviews or newspaper articles—when I get an opportunity to throw in some of the things we've learned in that inquiry, well I do. So it's sort of use it as an underlying subtle message that we need to be thinking about it all the time. And I'm hoping that the fact of my own weight loss [will help with that]. And, you know, I'll throw that in by talking about that as an introduction to a radio interview saying, 'well when I was out doing my morning run this morning it was pretty nippy', something like that, so that … to keep reinforcing the message of the regular exercise type thing. (Interview with an Australian politician, May 2011)

It is worth noting that there are a small number of proponents of the Nanny State narrative who draw on their personal experience to disparage obese individuals or reinforce a sense of 'fat blaming'. One author of an opinion piece in the *Australian*, for instance, noted mockingly of his own weight loss:

It was a miracle because it happened without the assistance of a Federal Government-sponsored obesity awareness campaign to spur me into action. I began to find myself in smaller clothes, even without a bevy of state premiers wagging their fingers at me and urging me to slim down. I slept better at night, despite there being no ban on fast food television commercials. My mood improved, even though I hadn't been motivated by an episode of The Biggest Loser with its avalanche of stretch marks. I did it by eating sensibly. By rediscovering exercise. By cutting back on the booze. But most of all, I did it by taking responsibility for myself.

There are perhaps hints of similar, though markedly scaled down sarcasm in Lord Nigel Lawson's comments to his peers in the House of Lords:

My Lords, as someone who has been there and done that, and indeed written a book about it, may I say to the noble Earl that he is absolutely right that this is not something that the Government can do on their own—indeed, may I suggest that it is not something that the Government can do at all? There is a genetic element, which the Government cannot do anything about, and the rest is about eating less and drinking less. (House of Lords, October 19, 2011)

On the very margins of this political debate, there are also some Role Models for precisely the opposite behaviour—champions of the Moral Panic narrative who challenge the characterisation of obesity as a problem. These are actors who embody obesity with comfort and pride. As discussed in the previous chapter, there is media coverage of social activists who embrace their obese bodies and represent them with subversive humour. But the influence of such actors is limited purely to the margins of (often voyeuristic) press coverage and does not penetrate expert or elite settings of policy discussion.

The Carer

More commonly in elite settings, advocates of Moral Panic do not embody the issue and they therefore represent knowledge on obesity in a quite different way. Next best to having 'been there' oneself is seeing obesity close at hand: as such, many elites present themselves in the role of Carer for the obese. Unlike with the Role Model, the prospect of redemption here is seldom predicated on the latent agency of obese individuals. These individuals remain passive recipients of treatment; it is, instead, the role of the Carer to take on the responsibility of protection. What remains at stake within this claim is the characterisation of that treatment. For Carers who subscribe to the Moral Panic narrative, obese individuals are targets and therefore victims of medical and policy intervention.

But, given the marginalised status of the Moral Panic account, the most prominent Carers in Australia and Britain are advocates of the Individual Intervention narrative. Their characterisation is obviously much more positive—obese individuals in this sense are beneficiaries of the support and diligence of professionals and practitioners.

At its heart, this claim rests on emotive appeal; the Carer's unique professional experience gives them empathetic insights into the challenges and experiences of obesity. One physician and proponent of the Individual Intervention narrative, for instance, explained:

[In my practice] I've just observed a common theme after common theme that was not being supported by other health professionals, or the government, or anyone. And it seemed to be that thousands and thousands of patients were feeling disempowered in this area of health, not knowing what to do, feeling that they had kept failing, feeling ashamed of themselves. (Interview with an Australian physician, July 2011)

A counterpart in Britain expressed his exasperation at the current model of funding for primary care which dehumanises the experience of obesity for patients, and disincentivises the pursuit of the preventative treatment that they badly need:

As a GP, I [generally] get paid based on the evidence, on the statistics, on how well I'm managing my patients' blood pressure. [But] for obesity, I'm given an incentive to count the number of fat people on my list, and then do absolutely nothing with that list of fat people, except a year later I weigh them again to make sure they're still fat enough to stay on my list so I keep getting paid for it. (Interview with a British physician, January 2012)

Likewise, an allied health professional in Australia emphasised the point passionately in her testimony to MPs at a public hearing for a Parliamentary Inquiry:

By the time the average patient gets to an [Accredited Practising Dietitian] they usually have been on a number of fad diets, shake diets, detox diets or tried to 'blast the fat' from their bodies—or simply have just stopped eating. They have been on a journey of erratic behaviours, frustration, anger and misery. Often they are simply confused. I see these patients every day. They are annoyed. They are annoyed at the 'bush doctors' and the conflicting, confusing advice and it often takes me one session just to have them regain some confidence in science and the healthcare system. (HoR Inquiry, September 12, 2008, pp. 19–20)

Indeed, the emotional attachment that Carers feel for the obese people in their care also makes them fiercely protective about remaining sources of 'fat discrimination'. One British physician, for instance, explained that it was the pervasive stigma associated with obesity that motivated him to move into public advocacy:

I was very concerned that the message in the media should be constructive. When I became involved, it was very voyeuristic. You know, articles in the newspaper, 'Big fat man, isn't it horrible? Isn't it amazing that he can't get out of his house because the door's too small?' I wanted to kind of redress the balance. So apart from quality and trying to get a scientific opinion included, I also started to work with more popular media—TV and radio and newspaper publications—to make sure they had a balanced view as well. Actually, we shouldn't underestimate the power and influence of the media on normal people. It's really important that, as well as talking to our patients in the consulting room, they're reading the right sort of information in the press. (Interview with a British physician, February 2012)

For these actors, their source of legitimation—the key thing that empowers them to speak on behalf of the obese—is the closeness of the relationships they have with obese people. One physician, for instance, became very animated in working to reject the notion of an 'obesity myth'. The essence of his claim was his proximity to the problem. For example, he suggested of Paul Campos (2004), the author who has popularised this account:

I think people who write such bollocks really need to look at the evidence and spend a day with me in my clinic on a Monday morning. I do clinics but also bariatric clinics in the bariatric surgery unit and my patients are getting fatter and fatter and they're getting more and more conditions such as Type Two Diabetes, which is more and more difficult to control. And then in the bariatric clinic I'm seeing the most horrendously complex cases you could possibly imagine. So, bless him, he's written a book and he's trying to sell a few copies and it's a novel and interesting argument that is just wrong. (Interview with a British physician, January 2012)

But this sense of proximity extends beyond a professional–client relationship. Some academics who conduct large-N epidemiological studies present themselves as 'close to the ground' and in tune with the emotional needs of the population that they research. One Carer who subscribes to the Moral Panic narrative, for instance, explained:

I think that was the first study to say, hang on a minute, this looks like social class stratification; hang on a minute, this looks like it might be ethnic. Because I went out to all of those schools myself as a researcher. I went to every one of those 35–40 schools. I was involved in measuring their heights and weights. And I could see the social class differences. And I could see the ethnic influences. Because I was out there at the coalface. I wasn't in my ivory tower. I think that's really important, to actually get out there and actually see it for yourself. (Interview with an Australian public health researcher, June 2011)

Carers feel they can represent the obese because they *care*.

The Nanny

Many of the other elite advocates in this issue area put themselves in the shoes of the Nanny. Nanny in this sense recalls stern oversight of the individual's best long-term interests, rather than tender affection—this is Nanny in the sense of the stern Victorian governess, not Mary Poppins.

Of course, Nanny is a loaded term in this context (see Chap. 4, Boswell 2015 and Swinburn 2008). As alluded to in the previous chapter, many elite actors are convinced that it is the damaging image of the Nanny State which stops them from mobilising public opinion effectively. My intention is to play off, rather than fully invoke, this common refrain. As such, my aim is not to critique these actors for adopting this role (especially not in the acerbic sense with which this term is often deployed in political debate), but to reflect the nature of the representative claim that actors in the public health lobby convey. It is the image of the Nanny—as determined to advance the broader interests of those they seek to help in spite of the lack of immediate appreciation that such a stance engenders—that best encapsulates the way in which proponents of the Social Dislocation and, especially, Structured Opportunity narratives work to speak on behalf of the obese. Indeed, some in the latter camp themselves are beginning to reclaim or rework the term 'Nanny' in order to subvert accusations of paternalism. One, for instance, reflected ruefully on the shallow arguments mounted against the banning of junk food advertising on children's television: 'Aren't nannies meant to protect children anyway?' (Olver 2008).

In contrast to the Role Model, the Nanny shows a deeper apprecia-tion of the structural obstacles that prevent individuals from exercising agency. Obese people, in the Structured Opportunity account, are vic-tims who are themselves, for the most part, powerless to affect change in the context of the 'toxic' or 'obesogenic' environment that they inhabit. One professional group representative in Australia explained, in reference to Role Model *par excellence* Tony Abbott:

[Abbott] is a fabulous role model in how he deals with those things. He's an extraordinarily fit man physically for his age and to be admired. But having had all the advantages. He has the time. He can buy the good bike. He can buy great running shoes. More importantly, [he doesn't have to] come home from work with the three kids and no help, just exhausted. (Interview with an Australian professional group representative, April 2011)

Moreover, while the Carer's claim is founded on emotional connection enabled by proximity, the Nanny's claim is founded on cold calculation performed at a distance. They see themselves as the true guardians of 'EBPM'. The crucial point is that Nannies see the bigger picture; that the individual challenges of obesity sit within a broader framework of environmentally or (especially for proponents of the Social Dislocation account) socially determined ill-health. A British public health academic went to great lengths in our interview to contextualise obesity in this way:

The whole notion is driven by fossil fuel mobility and the lack of exercise being built into daily life. It's also built into the ubiquity and the avalanche of calories that hit us. The shift in sizes. The shift from water to soft drinks. The sweetening of diets. And here we are with biology fixed 3–400,000 years ago. As the great Australian, actually a Kiwi, Boyd Swinburn based at Deakin, has endlessly argued and rightly so in almost everyone's view, the bodies are in the wrong environment. Environment is the environment as in built environment, there's that, but also the mental environment, the way we think, the ubiquity of messages. (Interview with a British public health researcher, February 2012)

But as well as this big picture, the other key component to the Nanny's claim is the distinct lack of reward they receive for their sober stewardship. This is especially prominent among proponents of the Structured Opportunity narrative. Unlike the well-resourced, well-networked, and, above all, well-remunerated representatives from the medical and food industries, their advocacy is a labour of love. One politically active Australian public health academic explained:

> The stuff I do in advocacy is not my day job. This is all done kind of as an addition. So my day-job is in research. The role I have taken since I've been involved in this is one of the advocate ... [who is] calling for change. We don't have that many levers being public interest advocates. We have tiny bits of money. We have tiny bits of time. We have no open doors to go knocking on. (Interview with an Australian public health researcher, June 2011)

Moreover, like the stern Victorian governess of popular imagination, they seldom feel the 'warm fuzzy' of appreciation. This was perhaps best encapsulated by a more junior public health professional in her appearance at a public hearing:

> I would like to think that there are some people in [an MP's] electorate who are alive today who would not otherwise have been unless we did some of that [population-wide intervention], but they do not know me and I will not meet them, and they will not send me a bottle of whisky at Christmas time thanking me for saving their life. That is how public health works. (HoR Inquiry, November 6, 2008, p. 47)

Knowledge, Agency, and Affect

The representative claims outlined above—as Role Model, Carer, and Nanny—all invoke a great deal of sympathy for the plight of obese individuals. They are avowedly rooted in compassionate interpretations of obesity as a public problem rather than as a private moral failing. Yet there are problems inherent in positing obese people primarily as passive or unwitting victims.

Firstly, coupled with the almost complete absence of obese actors from the debate—on the grounds that being obese would betray a hypocrisy or lack of credibility—such characterisations serve to undercut the sympathetic account of obesity that these actors are advocating for, regardless of their preferred narrative. Though portrayed empathetically, obese individuals remain, by implication, weak and incapable; they cannot speak for themselves in policy debate just as they cannot act for themselves to address their weight and health. A *Sydney Morning Herald* review of the Weighing it Up Inquiry, for instance, condescendingly acknowledged the poignancy of the handful of submissions from obese people. This acknowledgment served primarily to undercut (or blatantly poke fun at) these individual accounts:

> The three most moving submissions to the inquiry were from "Name Withheld". Each was from an obese person and detailed the causes and effects from their viewpoint. One blamed "brainwashing" of children. Another ("I eat when I'm hungry, angry, lonely, tired, even happy") blamed advertising and food labelling. And the third ("we are broke") argued that $100 a month to cover gym and weight-loss program expenses would sort the problem. In a wonderful non sequitur, Brian and Linda ("my wife and I are overweight") argued that "we find that bread also spoils quickly".
>   It's touching. But to state-fund? (Farrelly 2009)

Indeed, as this would suggest, the representative claims expressed by elites reinforce the stigma of the older account of obesity that they seek to displace. An opinion piece advocating for the Social Dislocation narrative in the *Guardian* explained the point thus:

> There's another government initiative on food, one more step in the process of raising awareness about what is really in what we eat. But I wonder whether anyone who is fat, or who lives with someone who is fat, really thinks it will matter a row of tinned flageolets ... Maybe there are other reasons for being fat but, in my experience, the most important factor is self-esteem ... Of course you know you shouldn't [binge eat]. But when every time you turn on the TV there's another solemn face telling you that being fat makes you a bad person. So who wouldn't? (Perkins 2008)

Secondly, speaking on behalf of the obese, however sympathetically, inevitably leads to the omission or glossing of key substantive issues and concerns. This is consistent with the philosophical claim for descriptive representation: the politics of presence enables a powerful reproduction of concerns and ideas rooted in lived experience that would otherwise be overlooked (see Phillips 1995; Mansbridge 1999). Take, for instance, the debate around food labelling. Typically, this discussion is framed in terms of evidence on psychology and consumer behaviour. However, one of my interview participants (a sympathiser of the Moral Panic account) pointed out the crucial human dimension that was lost in this narrow focus—that the imposition of traffic light labelling or any other such scheme risked reinforcing the shame and low self-esteem associated with obesity. Her point was that this prospect was being completely over-looked because obese people were not actively engaged in the debate.

Thirdly, and perhaps most importantly, even when substantive concerns are recognised and advocated for, the effort to speak for rather than with or to obese actors omits a powerful force that might act to more fully buttress the sympathetic account of obesity: emotional appeal. This links to some of the most important developments in interpretive and critical policy studies in the last decade, which have sought to emphasise the crucial role of emotions in policy discourse and political action (see Newman 2012 for a discussion; or, e.g. Larsen 2010; Durnova 2013). Of course, emotion is a key component of some representative claims made by elite actors, especially those who posit themselves as Carers. But the second-hand recounting of other people's challenges and experience, however credentialed, cannot match the effect achieved through first-hand testimony. One Australian politician shared that the most memorable experiences in her career—the ones which most motivated her to act—were interactions with the most affected members of the public. She explained:

> If, you know, you thought [a parliamentary inquiry on obesity] is going to be about diets and exercise, and then you look at a family where their kids are very large, and they pour their heart and soul out about the fact their lives have been destroyed by the bullying, the isolation, the sense of hate, and then the parents have this sense of guilt that they haven't been able to

help their kids. I mean, to hear people tell you those things, and to genuinely know the impact it's had on their lives, that must have an impact, I think. You're desperate to try and find a way that you can support them. (Interview with an Australian politician, June 2011)

Likewise, one of the members of the HoR Committee explained that the most affecting experience for him during the whole process was a casual encounter with a member of the audience during a break in proceedings:

I realised the emotional effect of obesity after a few loose comments that I made at an inquiry in Lake Macquarie where one of the members of the audience took deep offence. So it made me realise the mental effect … the way it affected people. (Interview with an Australian politician, May 2011)

Indeed, this was resolutely on display in the testimony of the only obese patient formally called on to provide testimony at the HoR Inquiry. This witness advocated through reference to her own personal story—an emotional account revealing deep personal hurt and struggle over years of weight gain, 'yo-yo' dieting, instances of discrimination, bouts of low self-esteem, and subsequent surgery and weight loss. She explained in response to a question about body image from a committee member:

I guess when you are really at your worst, when you are at the heaviest weight, you try not to think about your body image, because you are already feeling really bad and have a lot of psychological issues associated with being obese … [When you lose weight] you become quite obsessive about it. It is like, 'Okay, I only lost half a kilo this week. I am going to have to go harder.' Or, 'I have only lost one centimetre off my waist this week instead of two. What can I do?' You become much more compulsive and obsessive about it. That has huge consequences because in a way you become more self-loathing. You look at yourself and you think, 'How can I have gotten like this?' (HoR Inquiry, September 11, 2008, pp. 7–8)

Though out of step with the normal proceedings of such hearings, her advocacy came across as powerful and authentic all the same.[2] At the

---

[2] It is important to note that this witness's testimony came after her personal clinician had testified at a previous hearing, and it also preceded a string of testimony from experts and stakeholders later in the day.

conclusion of her opening statement, the chair of the committee made a special point of commenting:

> I would like to start off by congratulating you for telling us your personal story. I think it takes a lot to turn up and actually give us the very personal details of what you have been through. (HoR Inquiry, September 11, 2008, p. 3)

Though clinicians can go some way to replicating empathy through anecdotes about individual patients they have treated, their performances typically lack this raw emotive appeal.

Conclusion

This analysis has shown that the empathetic attempts to speak on behalf of the obese—be that as Role Model, Carer or Nanny—are problematic. Coupled with the steadfast emphasis on scientific evidence at the expense of, or at least in subordination of, personal experience, the effect is to reproduce traces of an older narrative on obesity which stigmatises the condition and those who live with it. In their effort to speak for obese individuals, these actors inadvertently work to delimit obesity as an elite, expert, and decidedly 'thin person's' cause.

Perhaps most crucial of all, then, is not just that elite representative claims reinforce 'thinness' as the normative standard, but that they stand in the way of broader mobilisation of public concern for the sorts of urgent policy reforms that, ironically, many of these actors devote their professional lives to promoting. One of my more reflective interview participants observed of the political debate on obesity in Australia:

> Standing on the sidelines [of the debate] to a large degree are the public because this is not an issue that people march in the streets for. This is not going to war. This is not cleaning up our environment. This is not AIDS or preventing road injuries or whatever. You don't see fat people with placards in the middle of the street. (Interview with an Australian public health researcher, June 2011)

This lack of mobilisation—mixed with a pervasive fear of the general public's (mostly) latent prejudices rooted in the older narrative of obesity (see Boswell 2015)—has served as a severe limitation in the call-to-arms of these well-intentioned advocates. It suggests that if campaigners on this issue really wish to promote and sustain impetus for policy action, they would do well to stand alongside, rather than in the place of, the most affected public.

References

Boswell, J. (2015). Toxic narratives and the deliberative system: How the ghost of nanny stalks the obesity debate. *Policy Studies, 36*(3), 314–328.

Campos, P. (2004). *The obesity myth: Why America's obsession with weight is hazardous to your health*. New York: Gotham Books.

Dixon, J., & Broom, D. H. (Eds.). (2007). *The seven deadly sins of obesity: How the modern world is making us fat*. Sydney: UNSW Press.

Dryzek, J. S., & Niemeyer, S. J. (2008). Discursive representation. *American Political Science Review, 102*(4), 481–493.

Durnova, A. (2013). Governing through intimacy: Explaining care policies through "sharing a meaning". *Critical Social Policy, 33*(3), 494–513.

Farrelly, E. (2009, July 18). The fat of the land. *The Sydney Morning Herald*. Retrieved January 15, 2013, from http://www.smh.com.au/opinion/the-fat-of-the-land-20090717-do52.html

House of Representatives (HoR) Standing Committee on Health and Ageing. (2008b, June 20). *Inquiry into obesity in Australia*. Melbourne: Hansard, Australian Government.

House of Representatives (HoR) Standing Committee on Health and Ageing. (2008c, September 11). *Inquiry into obesity in Australia*. Sydney: Hansard, Australian Government.

House of Representatives (HoR) Standing Committee on Health and Ageing. (2008d, September 12). *Inquiry into obesity in Australia*. Newcastle: Hansard, Australian Government.

Larsen, L. T. (2010). Framing knowledge and innocent victims. Europe bans smoking in public places. *Critical Discourse Studies, 7*(1), 1–17.

LeBesco, K. (2011). Neoliberalism, public health, and the moral perils of fatness. *Critical Public Health, 21*(2), 153–164.

Mansbridge, J. (1999). Should blacks represent blacks and women represent women?: A contingent "yes". *Journal of Politics, 61*(3), 628–657.

Newman, J. (2012). Beyond the deliberative subject? Problems of theory, method and critique in the turn to emotion and affect. *Critical Policy Studies, 6*(4), 465–479.

Olver, I. (2008, September 6). Curbing advertising will cut obesity. *The Australian*. Retrieved January 22, 2013, from http://www.theaustralian.com.au/news/health-science/curbing-advertising-will-cut-obesity/story-e6frg8y6-1111117397209

Perkins, A. (2008, January 24). Lose weight the self-respect way. *The Guardian*. Retrieved June 10, 2015, from http://www.theguardian.com/commentis-free/2008/jan/24/lostweighttheselfrespectway

Phillips, A. (1995). *The politics of presence*. Oxford: Oxford University Press.

Rail, G., Holmes, D., & Murray, S. J. (2010). The politics of evidence on 'domestic terrorists': Obesity discourses and their effects. *Sociological Theory and Health, 8*, 259–279.

Saguy, A. (2013). *What's wrong with fat?* New York: Oxford University Press.

Saward, M. (2009). 'Authorization and authenticity: representation and the unelected'. *Journal of Political Philosophy, 17*, 1–22.

Swinburn, B. A. (2008). Obesity prevention: The role of policies, laws and regulations. *Australia and New Zealand Health Policy, 5*, 1–7.

6

Claiming Knowledge

The almost complete absence of obese voices on this issue, as outlined in the previous chapter, was overall the most surprising and noteworthy reflection from my analysis, but it was not the most immediately striking feature of the debates in Australia and Britain. What took that mantle was the overwhelming 'fetish' for evidence and 'EBPM'. The debates in both Australia and the UK are saturated with references to these terms. Regardless of who they are or which narrative they adhere to, actors engaged in debate on this topic invariably stress the importance of scientific evidence in the abstract and make a point of basing their advocacy efforts on such evidence in practice. Indeed, though in Part 1 of this book I outlined the wide-ranging discrepancies among competing narratives on obesity, with significant contestation about the degree of individual agency associated with this problem, the scope of the problem, and even the existence of the problem altogether, there remained one common point along all this contested ground: belief in the 'evidence'.

The tendency among critical public health scholars has been to interpret the heavy emphasis on EBPM as an effort to 'depoliticise' the issue. The concern is about expert overreach and the attempted use of evidence

© The Editor(s) (if applicable) and The Author(s) 2016
J. Boswell, *The Real War on Obesity*,
DOI 10.1057/978-1-137-58252-2_6

to trump the democratic process (see Gard and Wright 2001; Campos 2004; Botterill 2006; Oliver 2005; Botterill and Hindmoor 2012; Saguy 2013). These scholars see the furore about obesity as a case of techno-crats abusing their status to advance their personal values and interests. Such an orientation echoes broader opposition to EBPM among critical policy scholars more generally, who interpret the recent focus on science in policymaking as an effort to reinvent the ill-fated rationality project in the governing of public affairs, and in the process enable technocratic elites to illegitimately dominate democratic politics (see Schwandt 1997; Parsons 2002; Roberts 2010).

In this chapter, I hope to show that this interpretation with respect to the obesity debates in Australia and the UK retains a small nugget of truth, but remains much too stylised and simplistic. I find that the overwhelm-ing emphasis on evidence does not prevent non-technocrats from engag-ing in debate, nor does it exclude other important sources of knowledge. Indeed, I reveal that actors of all types engage with the scientific evidence on obesity, that most have a sophisticated and reflexive understanding of the nature and role of evidence, and that they invariably weave claims based on the science together with other forms of knowledge, including personal experience, professional practice, and common sense. All this is not to say that I find the overwhelming emphasis on evidence entirely unproblematic: I conclude by showing how the hegemony of 'evidence' more subtly limits debate on this issue by further suppressing the emo-tional or affective side of this debate. Yet the overall message, picked up again in the conclusion to the book, is that the apparently universal com-mitment to EBPM need not necessarily be seen as an anti-democratic force of depoliticisation.

To build this argument, I focus firstly on the critical opposition to EBPM, both generally and in relation to obesity. I do so with a view to, secondly, outlining my empirical analysis of who engages with scientific evidence, how they do so (and how they reflect on doing so), and what effect the primacy of evidence has in debate. I conclude by consider-ing the implications for democratic contestation on obesity, laying the groundwork for the subsequent chapter that systematically analyses the manner in which knowledge claims are contested.

EBPM as a Depoliticising Force?

The New Labour government's commitment to implementing 'what works' in the late twentieth century saw a significant rise in interest in the concept of EBPM. Drawn from the terminology of evidence-based medicine (EBM) still dominant in health discourse (more of which later), EBPM was presented as being about pursuing policies based on their scientific credentials rather than on ideology or perceived common sense. Though some in the policy studies literature greeted this shift enthusiastically (e.g. Davies et al. 2000), the greater bulk have been more reserved. Some, especially influential scholars of a critical orientation, have been outright hostile to the cause of EBPM. For these scholars, EBPM represents an effort to 'depoliticise' key governance issues—to present them as technical matters of more or less certain fact rather than treat them as matters of ambiguous meaning or conflicting values (Schwandt 1997; Parsons 2002). EBPM is, in this view, indicative of the pervasive 'logic of discipline' whereby technocratic problem-solving displaces democratic contestation in the governance of public affairs (see Roberts 2010).

Traces of this broader critique of EBPM are apparent in the more sustained treatments of the obesity debate. Authors with a broadly similar critical orientation, writing for a variety of academic and public audiences, have taken issue with the obesity 'myth' in the Anglo sphere. This is the perspective that underpins the Moral Panic narrative identified in Chap. 4. In this scholarship, technocratic experts on obesity are presented as constructing this public health crisis. They are seen to be attempting to bypass the democratic process and 'depoliticise' obesity as a problem that ought to be tackled through expert intervention (Gard and Wright 2001; Campos 2004; Oliver 2005; Botterill 2006; Saguy 2013). The implication from this body of scholarship is that the overwhelming emphasis on evidence that I observe in Australia and the UK is indicative of a dangerous depoliticisation of this issue.

However, as I show in my analysis, such an interpretation is overly simplistic, failing to account for the complexities and nuances of knowledge claims made in these debates. Certainly, the 'fetish' for evidence with respect to obesity does condition and in important senses limit democratic debate on this topic—and I will focus on these limitations in the latter part of my analysis. But more broadly my analysis reinforces more recent scholarship in highlighting more equivocal implications for the debates in both Australia and the UK. I show how scientific evidence is increasingly becoming a common resource in democratic debate, reinforcing scholarship in science and technology studies which stresses the variety of actors who now routinely engage in interpreting and leveraging scientific evidence (see especially Hess 2004). I reinforce recent scholarship on the reflexive relationship between knowledge and policymaking by showing how the actors involved in debate are deeply thoughtful about the nature and role of scientific evidence in democratic governance (see Lahsen 2008). And I reinforce recent work on the complex politics of EBPM by showing how the use of evidence in debate inevitably becomes linked with, and mediated by, ideas, values, experience, and common sense (see especially Smith 2013). All of this challenges the reductive depoliticisation thesis and goes some way to explaining the intensely political contestation over knowledge on this issue, which is the focus of the following chapter. Before outlining this contestation, however, it is first incumbent on me to demonstrate the three claims made above.

Evidence as a (Somewhat) Democratic Resource

The depoliticisation thesis presupposes that scientific evidence is the domain purely of technocratic experts. And in some respects, to be very clear, this remains accurate. Lay actors, or actors engaged because they bring other resources to bear on the issue, are clearly less capable of producing and publishing compelling scientific evidence. While there are innovative efforts afoot elsewhere to democratise the production of science,[1] certainly that remains the case with respect to the data at hand on the issue of obesity in both Australia and the UK. A British health

---

[1] Examples include burgeoning work on 'science shops' that bring researchers together with civil society groups to solve pertinent practical questions (Leydesdorff and Ward 2005), and citizen science initiatives that actively engage citizens in the production of scientific knowledge (see Franzoni and Sauerman 2014).

charity representative, for instance, encapsulated the thoughts of many of my interview participants (from across a range of narratives) in expressing his cynicism about the influence of Big Pharma's money on the production of relevant scientific evidence:

> And they say they want randomized control trials. Well, who can afford to do them? (Interview with British NGO representative, March 2012)

Nevertheless, in important respects the interpretation and use of such data are now very much in the public domain. I find that virtually all actors engaged in debate across Australia and Britain, including those with no scientific credentials or claims to 'expertise', rely on and accentuate the importance of scientific evidence. Indeed, though the policy studies literature often casts researchers, practitioners, and bureaucrats as cohesive groups at loggerheads with each other, drawing on competing sorts of knowledge (e.g. Throgmorton 1991; Fischer 2003), my analysis aligns with scholarship which highlights the complex and imaginative ways in which scientific evidence is picked up and used by a multiplicity of political actors (see Hess 2004). So the focus on evidence is not just true of researchers and public officials, of whom this might be expected, but of industry lobbyists, health NGO representatives, and politicians, too. In order to advance a compelling performance of a narrative, actors must be fluent in the scientific evidence surrounding the issue—a point which is consistent with scholarship outlining a major shift in the relationship between experts and the so-called 'lay' participants in health policy debate (e.g. Akrich et al. 2014; several contributions to Lofgren et al. 2011).

Nowhere is this better exhibited than in the coalition behind the dominant Facilitated Agency narrative. This is an account backed by some academics and experts within the bureaucracy, but it is also supported by a number of lay actors—politicians, celebrities, food industry representatives, community activists, and so on. All clearly demarcate and draw on evidence as a distinct and particularly important category of knowledge. Indeed, one actor reflected that it was essential to keep a grasp on the scientific evidence in order to address adversaries across different venues of deliberation:

[In the media] we can't get into some of the evidence behind some of the things we say other than perhaps as a bit of a passing comment, you know, 'independent research has shown …' We can't get into who and what. But then obviously when we're going to talk to government, or when we're going to talk to the Diabetes Association, then we're going to have a string of evidence behind us, because that's also what they're looking for. (Interview with an Australian industry representative, June 2011)

Of course, the actors joined in this coalition do not necessarily have the same motivations with regard to the evidence on obesity. For the academics and clinicians who support the Facilitated Agency narrative, their commitment to the evidence comes from their identity as experts. One explained of the programme she gave testimony on to the HoR committee:

[As a researcher] I would also add that it is one of the few programs that is evidence-based. We have the theory, we have gone out and tested it and we have come back and said, 'Here is the answer'. (HoR Hansard, Adelaide hearing, p. 13)

For the politicians and public officials who do so, evidence provides administrative defensibility (see Hood 1991). One suggested in a frank reflection:

There are some legislative options open to government, but the evidence on them at present is certainly not unequivocal enough for governments to say, 'Yeah, we'll do that and take the consequences'. (Interview with a British public official, June 2012)

For some of the celebrity adherents, appeals to the evidence buttress their fragile credibility. David Gillespie, the author of a best-selling diet book, explained:

This is not my theory … I am a lawyer, not a doctor …. But everything that is said in the book is backed up by peer reviewed studies. (HoR Hansard, Gold Coast hearing, p. 6)

The same is true of the other narratives on the issue as well. The 'public health lobby' of expert scientists and professionals who adhere to the Structured Opportunity account quite clearly support their claims with reference to the evidence. But so too do the few supportive politicians who advocate this narrative. Former Australian Greens Party leader Bob Brown, for instance, made scientific evidence the centrepiece of his call for regulation of food advertising in 2009. Other prominent advocates of this narrative, such as newspaper columnists and NGO representatives, also rely centrally on 'the evidence' to support their claims. For instance, one prominent journalist with clear sympathies for the Structured Opportunity narrative spoke critically about a sensational 'obesity-denying' report from a rival outlet:

> Has he looked at the evidence though? Has he seen the evidence about diabetes? I saw he wrote a piece the other day. I see he had a piece last week on chiropractors, too. Well, what does the evidence say? … You tend to look at the data as you've seen it and speak to the people who you trust. (Interview with an Australian journalist, July 2011)

The same is apparent in relation to the Individual Intervention account. Again, one would expect the scientists and physicians who support this account to have a good command of the evidence but more surprisingly other, apparently 'lay' advocates appear equally cognisant of the science of the issue. Indeed, what is especially striking about the performance of the one and only obese witness of the Weighing it Up Inquiry, referenced at length in the previous chapter, is that she was so conversant in the evidence surrounding obesity. She was able to pepper her harrowing, personal testimony with reference to evidence-based improvements in treatment and support that were lacking in her case.

Much the same is true of the Social Dislocation account, where the tendency is again to make reference to scientific evidence over and above other sorts of knowledge. Take, for example, *Guardian* columnist Polly Toynbee's reflection on the decidedly 'circumspect' policy claims of the Foresight report. She caps a long-winding account drawing on social or cultural knowledge of fat shaming and the (non-existent) impact of education campaigns on obesity with reference to the then cutting-edge research of influential *Spirit Level* epidemiologist, Richard Wilkinson:

> Revealing epidemiological research in Richard Wilkinson's *The Impact of Inequality* shows how being at the bottom makes people sick, prone to obesity, heart disease and diabetes. (Toynbee 2007)

Perhaps this dynamic is more noticeable still among proponents of the Moral Panic narrative. Scientific evidence—of the epidemiological as much as sociological kind—is of course at the heart of expert advocacy on this issue. One such expert explained her frustration with much of the fanfare surrounding the 'obesity epidemic' as stemming from other actors not being 'scientific enough':

> [Public health experts] weren't scientific enough. They weren't rigorous enough. It came too late. And the whole debate became very skewed by a very sort of narrow medical model that's even not based on proper science. I mean fatness is not measured by Body Mass Index. Most of our data is based on just a measure for weight and height, and so the BMI measurement is a huge flaw that wasn't discussed in the early days of the debate. So the debate took off, the policy debate took off. It just took off in the media.

But the other sorts of actors who support this narrative equally draw primarily on scientific evidence. The most prominent example in Australia was a lengthy magazine feature in the *Australian*. The feature begins as an emotional plea, based on the experience of a family, but quickly transforms into a dense discussion of facts and figures on obesity. In particular, echoing the quote above from the Australian researcher, the author of the feature devotes considerable (and highly critical) attention in particular to the science of the body mass index (BMI) that underpins so many claims about obesity and its prevalence in Australia and beyond (see Guilliatt 2009).

Even the Nanny State account displays this characteristic. The broader perception of most of the elite actors that I interviewed was that this narrative remains rooted in ignorant prejudice. Its proponents are seen as hostile to evidence. One critic explained:

Wagging your finger at people and saying you're a bad person just go and lose weight, it doesn't work on any sort of scale … [F]rom a public policy, evidence-based perspective, there's absolutely no value in that argument in terms of changing anything. And it's a very dangerous argument … because it can be used to shut down debate about what is of value and worth. (Interview with Australian health official, July 2011)

Another was more succinct:

I think one of the frustrating things for me is that everyone's got their own opinion on this issue. Everyone thinks they're an expert because they've got a mouth. (Interview with an Australian clinician, June 2011)

Yet in reality the point is not that advocates of the Nanny State narrative reject scientific evidence wholesale. It is more that they adopt an outsider status to interpret such data differently to the experts who produced them. They use the data to support entirely different conclusions (see Boswell 2014 for more detail on this case). Indeed, even some of the most acerbic proponents of this narrative went out of their way to summarise key scientific findings on obesity to substantiate their claims (e.g. Sammut 2008a).

The upshot is that the overwhelming emphasis on EBPM does not, as critics would contend, have a depoliticising effect that delimits obesity as a technical issue of concern only to credentialed experts. The multitude of actors engaged in this debate, including adherents to all of the key narratives, are equally adept at making use of the scientific evidence surrounding this issue to promote their preferred account.

EBPM as a Reflexive Practice

The depoliticisation thesis, applied to obesity or more broadly, also seems to presuppose an uncritical devotion to science on the part of the actors who promote EBPM. In fact, I found the complete opposite. It was on the topic of EBPM, more than any other, that actors were keenest to engage in considered reflection. Indeed, as I alluded to in the introductory chapter, the use and interpretation of scientific evidence was never something I set out to focus on. It emerged inductively as actors in debate, and my interview participants, continued pushing it so far to the fore that it became impossible to ignore.

A clinical researcher (and advocate of the Individual Intervention account) spent much of the interview sharing her uncertainty and frustrations with respect to EBPM, and in particular the way discussion about the evidence invariably degenerated into a contest among competing disciplines and specialisms (a theme I will pick up on in the following chapter). She concluded:

> I guess the trouble is with the committees I've been on, the government sort of selects experts to be on the committees, and each of them comes in banging their own drum. And so each of them is worried about protecting their own silo, their own funding to their own institution, promoting their own profession because they want to be seen as the leader within their own group, so they don't come to the table really as an objective expert, they come to the table with a duality of role—one wanting to be involved in the process, but secondly to maintain and maybe grow their own silo within that.

An Australian public official reflected that interpretations of evidence were so diverse that the notion of EBPM in relation to obesity was close to meaningless. She said sarcastically:

> I mean who doesn't want to do things based on evidence? We operate our daily lives based on evidence. I feed my kids Vegemite sandwiches because the evidence is that that's what they'll eat as opposed to ham sandwiches. We all operate like that. (Interview with an Australian public health official, July 2011)

But, again, it was not just classical technocrats who felt this way. The multitude of other actors who make sense and use of evidence on this issue were equally thoughtful. A community NGO representative in Australia explained:

Evidence is never purely objective. And the slipperiness between what is subjective and what is objective, we have to acknowledge that that exists. (Interview with an Australian NGO representative, May 2011)

And an industry representative was equally cognisant of the political limitations surrounding evidence. He explained:

Of course whenever industry does any analysis. It doesn't matter—we can have independent, third-party people do it. We can have well-recognized researchers and academics do our analysis for us … As soon as the industry does anything it's like 'oh yeah, right, you know, we're not necessarily going to believe everything you're going to say because you've obviously got a vested interested in it'. (Interview with an Australian food industry representative, July 2011)

What this quote hints at is a high degree of scrutiny and contestation over supposedly 'evidence-based claims'. The difficulty, which proponents of most of the different narratives concede, is that the evidence remains uncertain and ambiguous. Many were quick to draw parallels to smoking, which has many decades of mounting scientific evidence behind it. A proponent of Structured Opportunity explained:

In the meantime, sadly, we probably don't have 60 years to wait. It's a dilemma. And so as policy makers—whoever they are—you have to strike a balance between the urgency of the situation and the quality of the evidence you have to support it. (Interview with an Australian primary health-care advocate, July 2011)

By the same token, a supporter of the Moral Panic narrative opined the apparent urgency associated with the so-called 'obesity epidemic':

And in other fields of health promotion like tobacco control, we've had 30 years to develop evidence and test out interventions, and see what works and doesn't work, and see what transfers and what doesn't transfer. It takes 30 years. And they want answers to this health issue in 5. And that's not possible. (Interview with an Australian public health researcher, July 2011)

Perhaps, though, the collective reservations are best summed up in this quote from a British public health official:

> It is of course theoretically possible that you can draw evidence from these sorts of sources to derive and develop policy, and in principle there's no reason why that can't be done. But in terms of practical politics it's sometimes a very tricky thing to try to do, for several reasons. Firstly, in the areas of broad social policy, as against medicine, the application of the principles of evidence-based medicine is much more tricky. There are certain things you just can't do randomised control trials on and, in any event, even if you could, the kinds of answers it would give you wouldn't necessarily be very helpful or it would be unethical. So there are some parts of policy where it just isn't applicable. Second, the evidence is itself rather patchy across many areas of social policy, of public policy, of education policy, of defence policy. And the notion that you can get this sort of abstract, disembodied evidence trickle down to the decision-making process is unlikely. So one has to be I think slightly cautious about the idea. (Interview with a British public health official, June 2012)

This was from an individual who had, at the outset of our interview, introduced his professional role as being that of an 'evidence-based practitioner'. As important as what he says above is the way he said it. The given quote is, quite staggeringly, completely unedited. This suggests more than off-the-cuff ruminations. Clearly, this was an issue he had considered and spoken about at great length already. There is no better illustration, then, of how the commitment to EBPM, at least in relation to this issue, is far from an uncritical shift towards depoliticisation. Instead, it shows that the pursuit of EBPM in this case is a highly reflexive practice.

Evidence as Just One (Albeit Crucial) Source of Knowledge

So by now I have hopefully demonstrated that the apparent hegemony of EBPM in this debate in both Australia and the UK does not marginalise non-experts, and nor does it uncritically enable technocratic dominance or depoliticisation. The point I want to stress now is that the emphasis on evidence does not prevent other sources of knowledge from being valuable and valued contributions to political debate. In spite of the privileged status of 'the evidence' in this debate, this is far from the only form of 'policy-relevant knowledge' (Tenbensel 2006) that actors draw on. In other words, my analysis has revealed, and many of my interview participants were happy to verify, that other types of knowledge claims— from personal experience, common sense, and professional practice—are equally important in actors' efforts to underpin the narrative that they support. As many recent studies have shown, the evidence itself seldom points unambiguously to a particular policy outcome. It needs media-tion—through ideas, values, experience, and other knowledge claims (see Smith 2013). The process of advocating on a complex issue such as obesity is inevitably one of tying together knowledge claims on a range of issues and from a range of sources (Head 2010). To make sense of 'the evidence', actors need to selectively assemble different components, linking them together or augmenting them with anecdotes, professional expertise, conventional wisdom, and statements of belief. I will show in the next chapter, when I outline the contest over knowledge claims sur-rounding obesity, that different forms of knowledge tend to be related to different narratives. But for the purposes of this chapter it suffices to show that actors themselves were more than willing to reflect on the value of knowledge beyond the strictly scientific.

This was especially true for clinicians and clinical researchers, whose understanding of evidence was indelibly linked to professional practice and daily experience. One, for instance, reflected thoughtfully on her own willingness to buy into the evidence supporting the Structured Opportunity narrative:

> I've thought a bit about this myself, and why I hardly needed any convinc-ing. And I think it really is my work. My patients come from some of the most socially disadvantaged parts of Australia. I work in the major public hospital in our region. I see some very severely obese kids. And I've been working in the area for a long time, so I've actually personally seen the evolution. (Interview with an Australian clinician, June 2011)

In contrast, another clinician, who supported Individual Intervention, reflected on his professional experience as something that underpinned his divergence from the broader 'public health lobby' behind the Structured Opportunity account:

> See the thing with public health people is, I'm sure they're very well-meaning, but they're not at the coalface, so they haven't had the opportunity—and it's no disrespect to them—they haven't had the opportunity of seeing what's going on. They haven't sat down and talked over these issues again and again. (Interview with an Australian clinician, July 2011)

An Australian proponent of the Moral Panic narrative reflected on the importance of professional and lay knowledge outside the research world, and how it could bump up against avowedly evidence-based practices:

> [I told the Weighing it Up Inquiry] that the social determinants of health, and health literacy will give you the best bang for your buck. But I don't think they published that! And a lot of social workers and people working in that social sector—that sort of social welfare sector—they would say the same thing. The woman with 6 kids whose giving the kids sausages each night may be better off being given food stamps than given a hit over the head with the big stick, or a note sent home from school, saying the child is fat, which is what they do in some of the southern states in America, Mississippi, Alabama—a note gets sent home saying your child is fat. Then what? Are you going to help me, or are you just going to keep whacking me with this stick? (Interview with an Australian public health researcher, June 2011)

Whereas for other actors, the Moral Panic account fell down precisely because it seemed detached from the everyday reality of personal experience. An Australian clinical researcher (herself a proponent of the Facilitated Agency narrative) explained:

> Whether you want to read it on a published paper, or see it on the TV, but you walk down the street, you can't help but avoid it. You know the other interesting thing—I know all the stats and I know all the papers. It's been around in our area of work for over 10 years [but the more striking thing]

is when you watch old movies. When you watch old movies from the 1970s, they're all really skinny. And it actually strikes you. Gosh, there's not that many fat people. So I don't know how you can claim it's a myth, unless you can become adjusted to, 'this is an okay weight'. (Interview with an Australian health promotion expert, July 2011)

For Carers—especially proponents of the Individual Intervention account—it is professional experience that provides this background. One advocate explained that his inspiration for getting involved politically was not through engagement with the science of obesity (contra simplistic myths about the prevalence of evidence-based practice in medicine), but through experience in general practice:

> When I started to grasp that my patients ought to lose weight for the benefit of their health, nobody could really tell me how to do it. So I started to talk to the great and the good … the people who knew the science of obesity. (Interview with a British physician, January 2012)

And even supporters of the Social Dislocation narrative, whose Nanny identity, as we saw in the last chapter, is typically buttressed by a detached sense of distance, reflected that the evidence needed to be taken in the context of everyday experience. Felicity Lawrence's (2008) essay on Jamie Oliver's *Ministry of Food* series seamlessly sews together evidence from some of Britain's leading public health experts with accounts of the individuals at the centre of the show, and their poignant plight.

The overarching attitude was perhaps best reflected by a prominent Australian public health researcher and well-known advocate of the Structured Opportunity account. When asked to reflect on the prospects and desirability of EBPM around obesity, he drew on the example of his advocacy regarding the issue of banning the advertising of 'junk foods' to children:

> The way that evidence is used in policymaking, or should be used, is that the sum total of evidence is weighed up. So the strong evidence marketing influences decisions and influences children and their preferences and their consumption, the strong evidence that what is marketed is junk food, and strong evidence if kids eat more of that type of food they get obese, and the

parallel evidence that if you bring in restrictions on marketing that we've seen with tobacco and with alcohol it will reduce consumption—all of those things, in a court of law, would make a substantive body of evidence to say we should move on it, particularly when you throw in societal responsibilities for protecting children, and throwing in the ethical aspects. For me, it's an open and shut case, and for most Australians, it's an open and shut case. (Interview with an Australian public health advocate, June 2011)

For policy scholars there are clear affinities here with the pioneering work of Giandenco Majone (1989) on 'analysis as argument', whereby he draws an analogy between policy experts and attorneys. Both, he argues, present information in packages designed to be compelling—and being compelling in policymaking requires more than just scientific evidence.

Yet, the point remains that scientific evidence retains a privileged status in this debate in both countries. Other sorts of knowledge matter. Indeed, they are essential to underpin any possible resolution. But in order to create a compelling package, the universal commitment to EBPM means that any narrative needs to be presented most prominently in relation to evidence, as an evidence-based account. One policy official, and proponent of the Facilitated Agency account, explained the dilemma as follows:

I honestly think if you look back, some of the boldest moves in public health have been based on what would be regarded in purist terms as not the best evidence, but on hunches ... a very colloquial term ... based on hunches that have developed from years of experience and practice, which aren't going to be documented in a randomised control trial. It's a bit hard to sell that sometimes. So we'll just keep saying we're working on evidence, doing the evidence-based work. (Interview with an Australia policy official, July 2011)

Evidence as a Muting Influence

This chapter was initially set up against the 'depoliticisation' thesis in both critical policy and critical public health scholarship, and I have laboured so far to show how the emphasis on evidence does not negate political contestation over obesity in either Australia or the UK. However, I want to spend the last section of this chapter underlining a more limited form of depoliticisation that I have observed across both debates; a tendency— one which reinforces the absences of affective representation of obesity as discussed in the previous chapter—for the overwhelming emphasis on evidence to drown out or mute the emotional side to this issue, particularly in or near elite institutions of policymaking.

The point here is that the privileging of evidence subtly reinforces rational norms that have traditionally suppressed the expression of emotion. To be clear, many of the actors in my analysis are very emotional about the issue of obesity—they care passionately about this topic and are often deeply concerned by the status quo and frustrated by their inability to affect change. And they often express this emotion, and make overtly emotional appeals, in their public advocacy. But—foreshadowing the claims I will make in Chap. 8 about the moderation of critical knowledge claims across political debate—this emotional edge tends to drop off as they favour more calculating, rational rehearsals of their preferred narrative as actors move towards empowered institutions of decision-making. They tone down their claims out of a desire to better fit the norms of the site, for fear of being seen to lack credibility.

Indeed, one of my most memorable encounters during my fieldwork was with an Australian public health expert and important figure on many of the networked arrangements for the governance of public health. This individual is unfailingly moderate in his public advocacy. But in our private interview, he revealed himself to be deeply emotionally invested in the issue. He spoke of his immense frustration at having to always 'watch what I say' and be careful to never make emotive claims that could not be supported with appropriate evidence. The commitment to EBPM conditioned and restricted his capacity to provide a truly compelling 'package'. He reflected:

I'm careful not to criticise the government when I think that could be misconstrued. All the comments I made … well, [public health] people are saying 'well, why haven't you gone further?' This is a really difficult area. If you want to take on promotions, for example, you've got to take on the manufacturers, the advertisers and the media all in one fell swoop … I mean I take my hat off to (then Health Minister) Nicola Roxon. She's been incredibly courageous on the tobacco stuff, on the alcopop stuff. She's copped an enormous amount of personal flak. She's got to fight with her own party let alone against industry. And industry, well, industries, [they] are proving themselves to be very nasty vested interests.

The point is not just in terms of how actors conduct themselves, but more deeply about perceptions of what sorts of knowledge claims can be influential in empowered institutions. A good example relates to ongoing debates about proposed treatments for obesity. There is a deep concern—among both proponents and opponents of the Individual Intervention narrative in particular—that the emphasis on evidence in these spaces of debate in decision-oriented sites of discussion can crowd out knowledge claims based on personal and professional experience.

Here, then, we begin to see the particular benefits of my approach to understanding narratives of obesity as live acts, performed across debate, rather than as dead texts, static accounts captured as a snapshot. In Maarten Hajer's (2009) dramaturgical language, on which my approach leans heavily (see Chaps. 1 and 2), the emphasis on EBPM *scripts* the rules of engagement in restricted terms that do bear the hallmarks of the older rationality project in policy analysis; it sets rational discourse as the norm, and thus subtly conditions the advocacy of adherents to critical narratives on obesity, excluding certain sorts of claims and downplaying the lived experience of obesity.

This is not the inexorable 'logic of discipline', whereby the issue is completely removed from political arenas of contestation. It is a much subtler form of depoliticisation, in which the keenest proponents of policy change become complicit in the neutralisation of the issue. It is at once milder but more pervasive. It thus represents both a challenge and an augmentation to reductive claims about the depoliticising effect of EBPM in policy scholarship. This is a point I return to in much greater depth in Chap. 8.

Conclusion

First, though, is a summary of what has been covered here. The discussion in this chapter has shown that the universal emphasis on 'evidence' in the obesity debate is not a straightforward 'depoliticisation' of a complex issue. The commitment to 'EBPM' should not be simplistically interpreted as ignoring all other forms of knowledge. The facts on obesity do not, and cannot, speak for themselves. Plenty of my interview participants reflected on the importance of drawing together common sense, professional expertise, personal experience, and ethical claims to the good with scientific evidence to put together a compelling 'package'. All actors did so in practice when advocating their preferred narrative of obesity across sites of democratic debate.

The emphasis on evidence does not completely marginalise other sorts of knowledge, but it does reinforce rational norms and, in the process, work to sideline the emotive. This is not to say that debate is unemotional—many of those engaged in debate are viscerally passionate about obesity and the need to deal with it as a health and social problem. But by couching their claims in terms of evidence, and always subordinating or enfolding other sorts of knowledge claims within discussion of 'the evidence', they legitimate the veneer of a detached, rational policymaking process that downplays the emotional experience of obesity and its impact on individual targets of obesity policy. Coupled with the absence of the affective or descriptive representation of obese people themselves, outlined in the previous chapter, the effect is an elision or marginalisation of the emotional dimension.

The germane point to foreshadow here is that the dullening of emotion and affect plays a key part in neutralising obesity as a political issue. This is at once more nuanced but perhaps more important than the simplistic 'depoliticisation' thesis. The fetish for EBPM does not negate the prospect of debate, but it does condition and limit that debate in subtle but important ways—and ways that are only exacerbated in the context of complex contestation and abstract conciliation, to be uncovered in the penultimate chapter. First, though, I turn my attention to how adherents to key narratives on obesity transmit their knowledge claims to empowered sites of decision-making to influence policies and programmes.

References

Akrich, M., Leane, M., Roberts, C., & Nunes, J. A. (2014). Practising childbirth activism: A politics of evidence. *BioSocieties, 9*(2), 129–152.

Boswell, J. (2014). Hoisted with our own petard': Evidence and democratic deliberation on obesity. *Policy Sciences, 47*(4), 345-365.

Botterill, L. (2006). Leaps of faith in the obesity debate: A cautionary note for policy-makers. *The Political Quarterly, 77*(4), 493–500.

Botterill, L., & Hindmoor, A. (2012). Turtles all the way down: Bounded rationality in an evidence-based age. *Policy Studies, 33*(5), 367–379.

Campos, P. (2004). *The obesity myth: Why America's obsession with weight is hazardous to your health.* New York: Gotham Books.

Davies, H. T. O., Nutley, S. M., & Smith, P. C. (2000). Introducing evidence-based policy and practice in public services. In T. O. D. Huw, M. N. Sandra, & P. C. Smith (Eds.), *What works? Evidence-based policy and practice in public services.* Bristol: Policy Press.

Fischer, F. (2003). *Reframing public policy—Discursive politics and deliberative practices.* Oxford: Oxford University Press.

Franzoni, C., & Sauermann, H. (2014). Crowd science: The organization of scientific research in open collaborative projects. *Research Policy, 43*(1), 1–20.

Gard, M., & Wright, J. (2001). *The obesity epidemic: Science, morality and ideology.* New York: Routledge.

Guilliatt, R. (2009, May 8). Off the scale. *The Australian* Retrieved January 16, 2013, from http://www.theaustralian.com.au/news/features/off-the-scale/story-e6frg8h6-1225710631861

Hajer, M. A. (2009). *Authoritative governance: Policymaking in the age of mediatization.* Oxford: Oxford University Press.

Head, B. (2010). Three lenses of evidence-based policy. *Australian Journal of Public Administration, 67*(1), 1–11.

Hess, D. J. (2004). Medical modernisation, scientific research fields, and the epistemic politics of health social movements. *Sociology of Health and Illness, 26*(6), 695–709.

Hood, C. (1991). 'A public management for all seasons?'. *Public Administration, 69*: 3–19.

Lahsen, M. (2008). Experiences of modernity in the greenhouse: A cultural analysis of a phyisicist "trio" supporting the backlash against global warming. *Global Environmental Change, 18*, 204–219.

Lawrence, F. (2008, October 1). Britain on a plate. *The Guardian*. Retrieved January 17, 2013, from http://www.guardian.co.uk/lifeandstyle/2008/oct/01/foodanddrink.oliver

Leydesdorff, L., & Ward, J. (2005). Science shops: A kaleidoscope of science-society collaborations in Europe. *Public Understanding of Science, 14*(4), 353–372.

Lofgren, H., de Leeuw, E. J. J., & Leahy, M. (Eds.). (2011). *Democratizing health: Consumer groups in the policy process*. Cheltenham: Edward Elgar.

Majone, G. (1989). *Evidence, argument and persuasion in the policy process*. New Haven, CT: Yale University Press.

Oliver, J. E. (2005). *Fat politics: The real story behind America's obesity epidemic*. New York: Oxford University Press.

Parsons, W. (2002). From muddling through to muddling up – Evidence based policy making and the modernisation of British government. *Public Policy and Administration, 17*(3), 43–60.

Roberts, A. (2010). *The logic of discipline, global capitalism and the architecture of governance*. Oxford: Oxford University Press.

Saguy, A. (2013). *What's wrong with fat?* New York: Oxford University Press.

Sammut, J. (2008a, April 33). Healthy lifestyles are taxing for everyone. *The Australian*.

Schwandt, T. (1997). 'Evaluation as practical hermeneutics'. *Evaluation, 3*, 69–83.

Smith, K. (2013). *Beyond evidence-based policymaking in public health: The interplay of ideas*. Basingstoke: Palgrave Macmillan.

Tenbensel, T. (2006). Policy knowledge for policy work. In H. K. Colebatch (Ed.), *The work of policy: An international survey* (pp. 199–216). Lanham: Lexington Books.

Throgmorton, J. A. (1991). The rhetorics of policy analysis. *Policy Sciences, 24*(2), 153–179.

Toynbee, P. (2007, October 19). We need to start a social revolution by truly putting children first. *The Guardian*. Retrieved January 18, 2013, from http://www.guardian.co.uk/commentisfree/2007/oct/19/comment.children

7

Contesting Knowledge

If the concern among critical public health scholars, tackled in the previous chapter, has been about the inappropriate depoliticisation of the science surrounding obesity, then it is the exact opposite that has led many mainstream public health scholars to express cynicism about the prospect of 'EBPM' in this field. For them, we are more likely to witness 'policy-based evidence making' than 'evidence-based policymaking' (see Black 2001; Marmot 2004). The cynicism is that 'evidence' can mean anything that actors want it to; that, with the increasing politicisation of science, actors reach for convenient 'truths' to support preconceived positions; that evidence just represents one weapon (among others) in the political battle over policy outcomes in contentious and complex areas.

There are clear affinities here with a broader cynicism in mainstream policy studies about the prospect of rational policymaking. Where the critical orientation holds that fact and value, science and politics, are inextricably entwined (Parsons 2002; Colebatch 2009), the more typical view is simply that political actors manipulate science. In this account, facts are pure, but their political use is not (see Oreskes and Conway 2010 in general; or Botterill and Hindmoor 2012 in relation to obesity specifically). In this way, the mainstream public health understanding of

© The Editor(s) (if applicable) and The Author(s) 2016
J. Boswell, *The Real War on Obesity*,
DOI 10.1057/978-1-137-58252-2_7

the obesity debate gels nicely with a broader account about the so-called 'merchants of doubt'. Like the corporations seen to be behind climate change scepticism, for instance, these shadowy actors, sympathetic to or bankrolled by the food industry, seize on outlying studies, partially represent data, and exploit popular misconceptions of 'how science works' to oppose significant regulatory reform. They stand in the way of EBPM. And so the presence of broad competing interpretations of the 'facts' about obesity, outlined in the previous chapter, would for these scholars illustrate the inescapable manipulation of evidence for preconceived political ends.

What I hope to do in this chapter again is complicate this rather simplistic representation. I will present a more fine-grained analysis of how actors contest knowledge claims across debate on obesity which shows that they do not fall in together neatly behind a narrative, simply cherry-picking and arranging evidence to most persuasively underpin their case. In fact, I will show that the competing narratives are beset by significant inconsistencies, overlaps, and fuzziness as they are performed across settings in both Britain and Australia.

What emerges is less a clash of competing narratives that just manipulate facts in service of a better story, and more a haze of conflicting and conflicted knowledge claims, driven by divergent values, epistemological assumptions, and motivations. At a more fine-grained level, what I find in each narrative is not so much the coherent assembly and reproduction of 'facts' to weave together a cohesive narrative, but a messier process of ad hoc justification which takes many different and sometimes incompatible forms. I also show that assumptions about the simple manipulation of science pay insufficient attention to the blurry boundaries between different narratives. In particular, because some of the narratives in this debate are performed by such diverse coalitions of actors in such different ways, it can be difficult to determine which account actors are actually supporting. Indeed, I argue this is so much so that it can lead to confused identities. Actors who strongly identify or are identified with a particular narrative sometimes actually perform a competing account through their public and private statements, without others (or even perhaps themselves) always realising it. The resultant haze serves to confound and confuse debate.

And so, if evidence is the key weapon, then policy actors are inevitably, in their own terms, 'hoisted with their own petard'. It is, I suggest, the commitment to 'EBPM' that plays a key role in fracturing and fissuring the coalition behind each narrative, but also in presenting the veneer of conciliation and consensus across debate, and thus masking or obscuring crucial aspects of conflict. The contest over knowledge, then, is not the polarised battle that it is typically represented to be. But it remains problematic nonetheless.

Conflicting Accounts of the Facts

My analysis reveals that these accounts are underpinned by broad disagreements about what counts as important evidence, what counts as sufficient evidence for action, and what certain bits of evidence mean. Though this section will outline these broad differences, it is important not to overplay the degree of coherence within the narratives, as will become clear later in the discussion. For the sake of clarity, Table 7.1 summarises the typical accounts of 'the facts' on each of these dimensions. The primary purpose is to give readers a broad understanding of the types of knowledge claims put forward and the sorts of justifications typically associated with particular narratives on the issue.

What Facts Matter?

Obesity as a policy space involves 'facts' about rates of obesity, the health complications of obesity, the related burden of disease on the health service and society more broadly, the health and economic impact of population-wide regulatory measures around junk food advertising, food labelling, new urban planning and transport approaches, and tax and subsidy reform; the impact of health promotion activities such as social marketing campaigns and community-based programmes; and the impact of medical interventions, including models of care, bariatric surgery, drug treatments, and so on. In terms of scientific evidence, each individual performance of any of the various narratives draws from

Table 7.1 Typical accounts of 'the facts' in the obesity debate

Narrative	Scientific evidence emphasised	Other knowledge mobilised	Approach to the facts
Facilitated Agency People have forgotten how to lead healthy lifestyles due to big social changes so they now need help relearning the basics	Data on successes of community interventions and lack of data for population measures	Common sense about the impact of major social changes; personal experience of weight loss success	Incremen-talism
Structured Opportunity The obesity crisis is a direct consequence of industry excess and a lack of regulation	Data on rise of obesity and chronic diseases; 'parallel' data on success of population measures on other issues	Anecdotes about the pervasive junk food culture; common sense about industry's profit motive	'Learning by doing'
Individual Intervention The obesity crisis has generated millions of victims who need immediate and ongoing medical help	Data on rise of obesity and chronic diseases; data in the Cochrane and Campbell Collaborations[a]	Professional expertise about the challenge of rising rates of obesity and about success of particular treatments	The Gold Standard
Social Dislocation The obesity crisis is a manifestation of deeper social problems due to inequality	Data focusing on socio-economic status and its impact on obesity and other social problems	Personal anecdotes about modern poverty and its impact on the vulnerable	'Big picture' policy-making
Nanny State Rising obesity is due to state interference and a decline in personal responsibility	Data detailing failures of public health interventions on obesity	Common sense about self-interested human behaviour	Economic rationality
Moral Panic Obesity has been unreasonably constructed as a crisis by vested interests	Data on obesity plateau; 'fat but fit'; and rise in eating disorders	Personal anecdotes about human cost of the rhetoric around the 'obesity epidemic'	'Do no harm'

[a] The Cochrane and Campbell Collaborations are organizations which undertake and collate systematic reviews of the scientific evidence on topics in the social and medical sciences respectively. See: http://www.cochrane.org/; and http://www.campbellcollaboration.org/.

a range of disciplines, incorporating figures on the prevalence of obesity from epidemiology, the modelled costs to the health service and to broader society from economics, the related physiological impacts from medical science, and so forth. But, as I outlined in the previous chapter, it also depends on support from other sources of knowledge. There are a range of professionals working on obesity-related issues who bring their significant practical expertise to bear in policy deliberation, from general practitioners and bariatric surgeons to health promotion practitioners, allied health workers, psychologists, food manufacturers and retailers, advertisers, physical trainers, weight loss gurus, and many more. There is also a range of personal experiences that actors draw on, referring to their own weight gain and loss, or their experience as parents, partners, friends, or carers. And there is cultural wisdom about issues such as family dynamics, cultural mores, and leisure activities.

I will briefly run through each of the competing narratives on obesity and how adherents to these accounts tend to assemble 'the facts' to justify their claims. As will become clear in the following section, it is important not to overplay the degree of coherence within accounts and the clarity of the distinctions between them in these terms—in fact, the fine-grained analysis offered later suggests considerable murkiness in the justification of claims across the contest of narratives. However, a broad outline in this section will help to provide greater context to this later discussion.

Adherents to the Facilitated Agency narrative typically weave together 'the facts' in myriad ways. Some, in particular the politicians, health bureaucrats, and health promotion researchers and practitioners who adhere to this narrative, emphasise case studies of successful community-based interventions (see HoR Inquiry, November 6, 2008, p. 15). However, for other adherents to this account—notably the food and advertising industries—the emphasis is more on the lack of evidence surrounding this issue. In particular, they highlight inconclusive data in relation to many of the regulatory measures that their adversaries in public health (who are proponents of the Structured Opportunity narrative) put forward. One of my interview participants talked on this point at length, concluding:

Thinking about the things that mess around in this debate—[a fat tax], banning advertising, traffic light labelling, product reformulation—all of those things. They all have a place. But none of them—none of them apart from reformulation—has any evidence that it makes one speck of difference to obesity. It's true. None of them. (Interview with an Australian food industry representative, May 2011)

Proponents of this narrative also draw on diverse 'facts' from other realms of knowledge. Many are particularly keen to draw on common sense maxims about recent social changes which they hold responsible for rising rates of obesity. One British public health official, who spent much of our interview discussing the scientific data, actually justified many of his most controversial claims in relation to common sense notions rather than science. In explaining the causes of the obesity epidemic, for instance, he claimed:

[There have been] big changes in the way we live our lives, the way we travel, the way we work, along with an environment which is packed with easy options, and on top of that, with human behaviour being what it is, we will tend to take the easier options put in front of us. (Interview with a British public health official, June 2012)

Other proponents of this narrative point to individual success stories of weight loss to show that obese people can have agency over their own lives. For example, in giving testimony to the HoR Inquiry, the executives from Weight Watchers Australia actually invited along their 2008 'Slimmer of the Year' to share her personal story with the committee members (HoR Inquiry, September 11, 2008, pp. 35–37).

Adherents to the Structured Opportunity narrative typically cherish scientific evidence from epidemiological studies. They focus especially on data about rates of obesity and related chronic diseases, and the impact of potential regulatory measures on those rates. Belatedly, there has also been growing focus on economic studies that assess the cost–benefit ratios of particular interventions (interview with a British public health researcher, March 2012). However, due to a lack of reliable data both in epidemiological and economic terms on many of the key policy instruments associated with this narrative—including changes to tax and subsidy systems around food, restrictions on food advertising, and regulations on food labelling—adherents are particularly fond of calling on 'parallel evidence' from other issues such as alcohol and especially tobacco control. One interview participant explained:

> Where's the cost-effectiveness or effectiveness evidence that [population-wide measures] will make a difference to obesity? There isn't any, and there never will be. But what we know from what we call parallel evidence [is that] these are the approaches that have made a difference when dealing with other epidemics, that that experience can be lifted off and taken to obesity with a degree of certainty. (Interview with an Australian public health researcher, June 2011)

These science-based justifications are combined with other sorts of knowledge. For example, public health practitioners recount stories about interventions and programmes undermined by food corporations, while advocates in other spheres draw on examples from their own experience or that of their children to show how 'junk food' convenience pervades daily life. But perhaps the most central knowledge other than 'the evidence' to most performances of this narrative is the popular perception that the food industry is amoral and profit-hungry. It is regarded as 'common sense' that the food industry is out to maximise its profits rather than have the interests of the public's health at heart, and thus all their efforts on this front are seen as exercise in public relations.

For adherents to the Individual Intervention narrative, the emphasis is on clinical or biomedical research. Adherents to this narrative typically point to evidence gathered through the 'gold standard' in scientific research—double-blind control trials of particular interventions and treatments. They typically suggest that 'the evidence' shows that only medical interventions, especially bariatric surgery and treatment provided through multidisciplinary clinics, are effective in terms of reversing obesity (Proietto 2008; Campbell 2010). Advocates of this narrative equally stress the importance of professional expertise, particularly that of clinicians. Such is the importance placed on this knowledge that, in the only example in my analysis of an actor using the term 'evidence' to apply to anything other than data derived from scientific inquiry, one even referred to his clinical experience as 'a level of evidence' in discussing the issue (interview with an Australian clinician, July 2011).

Advocates of the Social Dislocation narrative tend to focus on epidemiological data. For these actors, the emphasis is on the socio-economic gradient in obesity, whereby those of low socio-economic standing have proportionally higher rates of obesity than those of high socio-economic standing. Advocates of this narrative are, more than anyone else in the debate, conscious of linking data about obesity to other social indicators such as unemployment, crime, and housing. Adherents to this narrative also typically draw on personal anecdotes of hardship and social dysfunction. Indeed, some of the most powerful performances of this narrative in the British media have involved focusing on obese individuals, families and communities, and generating a broader sense of empathy for their situation. The articles focusing on the single mother depicted in Jamie Oliver's *Ministry of Food* television series (Lawrence 2008), and the plight of nearly the entire population of an old mining town in Wales (*The Daily Mail* 2011), already discussed in Chap. 3, are two prime examples.

Advocates behind the Nanny State narrative tend to take a broad view of the scientific data, summing it up as evidence of a failure on the part of public health. In fact, many proponents see it as even worse than that. For them, it is not just that clinical and population health research has failed to stop the rise of obesity, but that it has actually contributed to it by dispossessing individuals of personal responsibility. One newspaper article began with a withering dismissal of public health research:

Excuses, excuses, excuses. Yet another excuse has been put forward to account for the epidemic of obesity in modern society. (*The Sydney Morning Herald* 2009)

While adherents to this narrative generally reject professional expertise as being driven by self-interest, they align scientific data with insights from common sense to present a coherent account. As this suggests, adherents of this narrative put particular emphasis on neoliberal assumptions about human nature and the tendency of individuals to be fundamentally self-interested.

Finally, advocates of the Moral Panic account draw across a wide range of scientific evidence on various issues. Many adherents to this narrative emphasise evidence about obesity rates, with heavy criticism of epidemiological studies extrapolated from current BMI assessments. Instead, there is much more emphasis on more nuanced measurements which, proponents of this narrative argue, show that obesity rates have largely plateaued or even declined (interview with an Australian nutrition researcher, June 2011). Many also draw attention to public health evidence showing that people can be 'fat but fit'—a theory that what matters for health outcomes is not your weight but how active you are—as a way of criticising the rhetoric around the 'obesity epidemic' (Aphramor 2009). And finally, some members of the ensemble behind this narrative also point to evidence about the increasing prevalence of bulimia and anorexia nervosa, tying this to the political and medical 'crusade' on obesity (Henry 2008).

Advocates of this narrative also draw on other sources of knowledge. They put special emphasis on personal anecdotes from individuals branded obese by practitioners and policymakers and the pain and anguish they suffer as a result. One article recounted the personal anecdote of a parent who was informed her daughter was 'overweight or at risk of becoming obese' by zealous health authorities:

> On one level this was absurd, for anyone could look at Bianca Stoneman and realise she is not even chunky, to use an old-fashioned term. But the more Jodi Stoneman read the letter ACT Health had sent her—with its warnings about the dangers of diabetes and high blood pressure, its links to the Westmead Children's Hospital website and its suggestion that she consult her doctor for advice about nutrition—the more confused and offended she became. (Guilliatt 2009)

What Do the Facts Mean?

In the section above, I have tried to show that proponents of different narratives tend to focus on different sorts of 'facts'. It is important to note, however, that there are some 'facts' that are widely considered crucial. Yet I find, in line with influential work on evidence and meaning in other policy struggles (Fischer 1995), that interpretations differ drastically even on these 'settled facts'. The clearest example of this, of course, is evidence about increasing rates of obesity, which all but proponents of the Moral Panic narrative accept is correct. Obviously, as outlined in Part 1, advocates of different narratives interpret this established 'fact' very differently. But the same point is also true of some of the smaller points of controversy around this issue.

One core piece of evidence nearly everyone draws on is data revealing that health promotion activities such as social marketing campaigns have had little or no demonstrable impact on obesity rates. For many of those who support the Facilitated Agency narrative, it is seen as a chance for policymakers to learn from past mistakes and develop an effective approach to educating the population. For example, one state public health bureaucrat explained in her testimony to the HoR Inquiry: 'We do have quite a lot of data about the effectiveness of this type of program and what you need to do with that' (HoR Inquiry, November 6, 2008, p. 8). For those who support the Structured Opportunity narrative, this evidence is typically seen as proof that such interventions do not work in our current environment—that they need to be allied to strong-armed regulation as part of the 'comprehensive approach' discussed in the previous chapter (interview with an Australian public health advocate, June 2011). For those who support the Individual Intervention narrative, though, this evidence simply demonstrates the futility of current population-wide strategies altogether:

> There are calls for massive public education programs on obesity, bans on junk food, restrictions on advertising and food-label reforms … But, sorry, none of them will work. (Proietto 2008)

For those who support the Social Dislocation narrative, it is further evidence that superficial policy measures cannot impact on such a deep-seated social problem (interview with a British public health researcher, 2011). For those in favour of the Nanny State narrative, it shows that government has little power to influence private matters in this way (Sammut 2008). And for proponents of the Moral Panic narrative, who challenge the notion of an 'obesity epidemic' anyway, it is evidence that all efforts on this front are counterproductive (Guilliatt 2009).

There is also major contention over the issue of restricting or banning advertising of unhealthy food products to children. Some even describe this as the key 'policymaking battleground' on obesity in Australia (interview with an Australian public health researcher, June 2011), though not everyone considers the facts surrounding this issue to be especially important. The scientific evidence on this issue is very limited. It has only been trialled in two jurisdictions for a sustained period—Sweden and the Canadian province of Quebec (for a background discussion, see Jolly 2011). Advocates of the different perspectives draw on the evidence from these cases in very different ways, allying it with other sorts of knowledge to create competing interpretations of whether or not the regulatory measure is a good idea. For advocates of the Structured Opportunity account, the evidence from these cases is considered promising, albeit tainted by some limitations in the way restrictions were implemented. Combined with 'parallel evidence' about the success of advertising restrictions on tobacco, and simple common sense, they suggest that the weight of evidence shows this is a good policy option. Indeed, one advocate concluded:

> I think tobacco advertising was banned in 1976. How good was the evidence then? Not great. But it makes sense. It's common sense that advertising affects demand, which affects sales, which affects consumption, which affects disease. (Interview with an Australian public health advocate, June 2011)

For advocates of the Nanny State narrative, though, the evidence shows that such restrictions make no difference to obesity rates and are fundamentally a waste of time. An editorial for the *Australian* (2008b) newspaper put it colourfully:

> In a free society in which advertising is part of life, banning junk food commercials, the clarion call of many dietitians and medicos, is futile and draconian. It would do nothing to teach people to make better choices when confronted with too many tempting options. Nor would such a ban help parents teach their children one of the most important words they need to hear in relation to lollies, junk food and, later, alcohol abuse, cigarettes and drugs. That is: 'No'.

Many of those who support Individual Intervention narrative in Australia have a similar interpretation, taking it further though to suggest that this is symbolic of the fact that population-wide measures cannot work. One confided in an interview that she dreaded going to committee meetings with public health experts who would always 'get the conversation stuck' on this issue: 'I don't care what they say; there is no evidence' (interview with an Australian clinical researcher, July 2011). Some who support the Facilitated Agency narrative adopt a very similar line. Other proponents of this narrative, though, do not draw on this evidence to dismiss the idea out of hand. Instead, to justify delaying action on this front they focus on pragmatic difficulties and scientific uncertainties experienced in the Swedish and Quebecois cases around defining and monitoring unhealthy foods. One explained:

> So even something as simple as saying let's ban advertising junk food to children gets you into a very technically complicated business of determining what junk food is on the basis of its nutrient content. And of course food manufacturers are always reformulating their products anyway for taste, shelf-life and all sorts of things, and because of that what is a junk food last week may actually fall the right side of the line next. So it sounds like a simple solution, but in fact it's not. From a government's point of view it's a regulatory nightmare. (Interview with a British health official, June 2012)

Another issue around which there is considerable contention over the meaning of stable, accepted scientific data is bariatric surgery. Most advocates of the Individual Intervention narrative point to empirical evidence from trials of this surgical procedure as proving its efficacy and cost-efficiency. In fact, for many proponents of this narrative, this evidence is the core of their account, and they make every effort to highlight its significance. Yet for adherents to other narratives, this evidence is not so compelling. Prominent advocates of the Structured Opportunity account, for instance, have voiced their concerns about calls for greater funding for surgical procedures:

> Lap-band surgery, while it may be suitable in some extreme cases, is a Band-Aid response. This new epidemic is our greatest public health

concern and we need a population-based public health strategy to beat it. (Zimmet and Jennings 2008)

As this indicates, most advocates of the Structured Opportunity narrative accept that evidence shows the procedure to be effective in certain circumstances, but they believe that granting greater access to the procedure is an inappropriate policy response to a population-wide problem. For advocates of the Moral Panic narrative, though, the evidence is actually deeply disturbing. It simply reveals the power of vested interests in medicine to fund research solely for the purpose of financial exploitation. In particular, they point to the human dimension lacking from the cold data on this procedure, drawing on harrowing personal anecdotes of pain and indignity which the surgery is allegedly responsible for. One adherent to this narrative explained to me in an interview:

> There's the whole sort of public debate on blogs from people that have had the gastric banding, and how much distress they've experienced, and they haven't had the support from surgeons that they've required, and that they've ended up feeling nauseous with heart burn and reflux, and how they've been sold the procedure but not the follow-up support. (Interview with an Australian nutrition researcher, June 2011)

How Should the Facts Inform Policy?

Finally, while adherents to the competing accounts use different sorts of 'facts' and interpret even similar 'facts' in different ways, perhaps the starkest distinction between the different accounts concerns their approach to the use of knowledge in policymaking. Although again there are important differences and inconsistencies within competing narratives which I will highlight later, there is a tendency for adherents to the same narrative to espouse the same sort of belief about how 'the facts' should inform policymaking around this issue.

The Nanny State narrative is typically underpinned by an economic rationalist approach to knowledge utilisation. Though not always spelled out in some of the 'lay' performances, such as in newspaper correspondence, adherents to this narrative often draw on the logic of the market as a way of explaining and linking scientific observations. They draw on assumptions about rational actors making calculating decisions. One proponent explained:

> Obesity is not a public health problem and should not be treated as one .... Britain's National Health Service shows what can happen when the government makes all health problems its business—[economic] calculations rapidly lose their compassion and become cruel assessments of moral, rather than medical, questions. (Berg 2008)

Those who support the Facilitated Agency narrative often reflect an incrementalist approach to policymaking (for a classic account, see Lindblom 1959). They emphasise the limited knowledge that policymakers have about this issue and suggest that in the absence of clear knowledge a relatively gradual introduction of measures and policies is a more justified course of action. One explained:

> I think we're really talking about a really long-term situation. It's going to be about incremental moves, and small increments at that. And those moves will have to come from all parties and a range of sectors. (Interview with an Australian health bureaucrat, July 2011)

In contrast, the more coordinated coalition behind the Structured Opportunity narrative tends to endorse a 'learning by doing' approach to the facts surrounding obesity. Indeed, this was the slogan running through the Taskforce's key report, which is held in such reverence by Australian proponents of this narrative. Echoing contemporary policy scholarship and its emphasis on the importance of 'policy learning' in real time (see Sanderson 2009), these actors suggest that action needs to be taken now in order to counter the threat of the obesity crisis. For them, reliance on watertight evidence stifles innovation and underplays the urgency of the situation (interview with a British public health advocate, March 2012).

Most proponents of the Individual Intervention narrative hold a zealous belief in 'EBPM'—a slogan used by all sides in this debate but with particularly positivist connotations in the hands of some adherents of this narrative. Indeed, many who subscribe to the Individual Intervention account demand that only evidence codified in the Cochrane and Campbell Collaborations is a suitably rigorous basis for policy action. One clinician explained:

> Well, I've always been brought up obviously as a physician to use evidence-based medicine. Every decision I put to my patients I must be able to back it up with the science that says I'm doing the right thing. I was surprised therefore when I learnt that politicians and policymakers don't have to do anything of the sort. They can just come up with the idea and implement it. It has come as a bit of a shock. (Interview with a British clinician, May 2012)

Adherents to the Social Dislocation account, on the other hand, typically approach the 'facts' with a much 'bigger picture' in mind. They draw on neo-Marxist ideas that it is deep social structures that cause and sustain such policy problems (see John 1998, pp. 93–100). For them, then, the 'facts' around obesity need to be seen in the light of the broader societal context in which they occur. Renowned expert Sir Michael Marmot, whose standing in this debate has already been touched on made this clear in his response to an opinion piece calling for more personal responsibility. He claimed that the 'evidence suggests that simply telling people to behave more responsibly is no more likely to be effective than telling someone who is depressed to pull his socks up'. Instead, he argued, it is incumbent to look beyond the behaviours and environments that lead to obesity and look to 'the causes of the causes', concluding that the 'behavioural choices we make as individuals are rooted in our social and economic circumstances' (Marmot 2010).

Finally, many adherents of the Moral Panic account support a 'do no harm' principle (O'Dea 2010). For them, measures introduced without a sound knowledge basis are not only unjustified—as adherents to the Facilitated Agency narrative would have it—but actually risky. They suggest that policy decisions made rashly could have negative ramifications later on for various actors engaged in the debate, most especially the obese people at the centre of it. One proponent of this view maintained:

> We are worried that things are going to be implemented without sufficient evidence to back them up. A couple of things can happen: you can spend a lot of money implementing an intervention and it can work as hoped; after the follow-up period you can find that there has been no change; or, the worst outcome, after the follow-up period you find that harm has been done. (HoR Inquiry, November 6, 2008, p. 28)

Conflicted Accounts of the Facts

There is a common presumption that political narratives represent neat, coherent assortments of knowledge claims.[1] This is a perception that equally carries through to political practice, and the actors I encountered in this study. Nowhere was this better exemplified than with the production of the Foresight report in the UK.

> Most importantly [the Foresight process] exposed how actually the obesity thinkers hadn't really got a good narrative. They hadn't got a concerted— and I used that word advisedly, concerted, brought together in some harmonious way—a concerted narrative of what to do. And [bringing together that narrative] was the most useful thing about Foresight, through our celebrated diagram of the 'obesity map' as it is now called. (Interview with a British public health researcher, March 2012)

But contra these assertions of unity and coherence, at a finer level of detail, I find that each narrative and coalition is far less cohesive than the initial analysis would imply. What I find is not so much united coalitions

---

[1] This presumption or emphasis on narrative coherence is apparent in much of the literature that lightly touches on narrative as a concept but is also central to some analytical accounts that focus on narrative in policy and political debate (see, e.g. Grube 2012; Jones and McBeth 2007). Yet, of course, some of the key pioneers of the narrative approach to understanding political debate long forewarned about the messy, ambiguous nature of narratives in public debate (see Stone 2002; Yanow 1993; Hajer 1995).

of actors assembling and reproducing evidence to justify agreed ends, but more disparate coalitions of actors who often draw on and emphasise different sorts of evidence in different, sometimes incompatible ways. These differences stem, I suggest, in part from material and disciplinary conflicts within these coalitions, but just as importantly from differing ideological and epistemological commitments.

Material Interests

In some cases, the cracks in the coalitions stem from material conflicts between members. Advocates of the Individual Intervention narrative, for instance, concur about the importance of greater investment in medical research and practice in general terms, but can have very different ideas about the relevance and reliability of the scientific evidence therein. Two proponents of this narrative that I spoke to—one in Australia, the other in the UK—were broadly positive about the evidence of efficacy of surgical procedures and pharmaceutical products in helping fight obesity. Another two—again one from each country—were pessimistic about the evidence, dismissively suggesting that pursuing surgical and pharmaceutical solutions was like trying to develop a 'magic bullet'. They instead promoted greater investment in 'coordinated care' for obese individuals. One of the latter explained about bariatric (weight loss) surgery:

> The results that I've seen are very poor ... At 6, 7, 8 years there's a gradual rate that people gain weight again. Some of the researchers who've looked at a run of lapband patients ... [say] we don't see the positive outweighing the negatives for these people because there's so much risk along the way. (Interview with an Australian clinician, June 2011)

The former pair stood to benefit financially and professionally from investment in surgical and pharmaceutical solutions; the latter pair from investment in 'coordinated care'.

Yet a cynical reading of such divergences on the evidence within coalitions stemming solely from material conflicts risks being reductive, not least because it is something about which most actors are acutely aware—especially clinicians and public health academics who have actual or potential access to pharmaceutical and medical industry funding. One reflected on the 'dilemma' this posed:

> [Pharmaceutical companies] threw an awful lot of money at promoting the concept of obesity as a disease because they were producing drugs to support treatment. I took that money and used it to fund an organisation ... When I stepped down from the organisation, I found that the pharmaceutical influence was considered to be detrimental and would impair my credibility. (Interview with a British physician, April 2012)

Fractured Identities

A second key point concerns conflicts among adherents to the same narrative based in divergent disciplinary commitments. At a broad level, as I have stressed in the preceding discussion, the various disciplines that intersect with the analysis of scientific evidence on obesity inform and align with competing narratives (e.g. epidemiology and the Structured Opportunity narrative; sociology and the Moral Panic narrative). But closer inspection reveals considerably more overlap, leading at times to visible fracturing in the identity of the actors involved.

Take, for example, the widespread effort made to better incorporate economic evidence and expertise by many proponents of the Structured Opportunity narrative. For some, this is seamless and necessary if public health experts are to maintain influence in policy circles. One explained:

> In the traditional scientific intervention—research intervention—health economics is sort of an add on or something you come to afterwards, if you think about it at all, rather than being one of the first things you embed right up front. Many of us doing research haven't actually done it with a policy focus in mind. We've done it because we're interested rather than because we're thinking 'how might this work if I did it', 'how could I make this relevant to policy makers', or 'how could I make it relevant to the community'? So actually ... [if policymakers] could see that it might lead to economic benefits, that's going to be very powerful compared to the

traditional randomised control trial with just one health outcome. (Interview with an Australian clinician, June 2011)

Yet, for others, health economics remains an alien and rival discipline, whose practitioners cannot be relied on as allies in political debate. Referencing a report on childhood obesity reduction initiatives produced by the Productivity Commission (a body that provides specialised cost–benefit analyses of policy interventions for the Australian government), one interview participant did not hold back in his condemnation:

> That was bullshit that article they put out by junior researchers! Did you see who wrote it? Well, go and have a bloody good look at it! It was utter crap! It was an extremely poorly researched and poorly put together paper, done by junior researchers that fundamentally have no idea what's going on and nor does the research. Why did they get away with it? I don't know. Ask the Productivity Commission. I mean it's a woeful piece of work. And that's why I wouldn't let economists loose in a paddock. (Interview with an Australian public health researcher, June 2011)

At other times, the disciplinary bond can seemingly obscure discrepancies in substantive interpretation. This was most clearly exhibited on a day when I was travelling intercity to conduct interviews with British obesity experts. At the end of an interview with a British physician, he spoke glowingly about an 'ally' who worked at a government agency devoted to public health—an expert who I was coincidentally scheduled to meet later in the day. However, while the physician was a passionate supporter of the Structured Opportunity narrative, the official in question—in both our interview and in his few public statements—is in my analysis clearly not. Where the physician openly vilifies the food industry and promotes regulatory shackles, his alleged 'ally' in formal governing institutions downplays the role of the food industry, cautions against the exaggerated claims of his colleagues in the public health community, and urges a slow, incremental, pragmatic, and collaborative approach to solving the obesity problem.

The broader point, then, is that disciplinary identities do not map neatly onto narrative identities. This can serve both to generate conflict despite substantive agreement, and to obscure conflict despite substantive disagreement—a point I will return to in some depth in the next chapter.

Ideological Commitments

Running deeper than mere material concerns or even disciplinary divergences, inconsistencies in the way actors draw on evidence can also relate to ideological conflicts or incompatibilities among proponents of the same narrative. Consider these two quotes from adherents to the Moral Panic narrative:

> (It may be) we've just reached a situation where we're so saturated with opportunity for inactive play, it's so easy to access energy-dense food, high-caloric food, that any child that will become overweight or obese has become overweight and obese. (Olds in Ryan and Bita 2009)
>
> I think people worry about health because it's the easiest place to hang fat hatred. The data actually suggests that it has to do with activity, and not size. (Allen in Cowell 2010)

Though often seamlessly encompassed within the same account (e.g. Guilliatt 2009), these claims are actually in conflict. For Olds, the public health expert, the key evidence is that obesity (in children) is not increasing. For Allen, the activist, however, Olds's interest in whether obesity is increasing is irrelevant, because the evidence suggests that size does not matter anyway. This hints at an uneasy alliance driven by different ideological commitments: in Olds's case, a conservative orientation to state interference in private lives; in Allen's case, a radical repudiation of a 'paternal' state and medical establishment.

The same sorts of ideological disjunctures are apparent in the broad coalition behind the dominant Facilitated Agency narrative and manifest in the way different sorts of adherents to this account understand the idea of an incremental approach to the use of evidence. For some, especially researchers and bureaucrats, incrementalism is a pragmatic move based on their assessment of the political context. One explained:

[Progress] can only happen in my view gradually because the political options that are available to government are really rather limited. Some progress has been made ... but there's a still a long, long way to go. (Interview with a British public health official, June 2012)

For others in this coalition, though, a commitment to incrementalism stems more from an ideological commitment to 'small government'. A food industry representative, for instance, argued:

Regrettably we come from two different philosophical points of view. You [Senator Brown] come from a regulatory point of view; wherever you see a problem you wish to regulate ... This industry is coming from the point of view that there is a problem and we will act responsibly to address that problem without the need for regulation. (Senate Hansard, Canberra hearing, 2008, p. 16)

Epistemological Assumptions

Discrepancies among proponents of the same narrative can also reflect deeper conflicts in epistemological assumptions, even where material interests and ideological commitments appear to align. This is apparent among the organised public health lobby that supports the Structured Opportunity narrative—a coalition of actors who have consciously worked to 'strengthen their hand' (interview with an Australian public health advocate, April 2011). Though most of these actors share the same material incentives (investment in research) and claim to share similar political ideologies (a lack of faith in free markets and an insistence on government interventions), some of the discrepancies in the way actors in this coalition approach and use evidence in this debate reveal deeper differences about what is actually knowable.[2]

---

[2] The conflicting epistemological assumptions on display in this analysis are typical of conflicts found within scientific communities. They reflect the different approaches that scientists take to issues of certainty and confidence, and how these manifest in the manner in which they engage in other venues of public deliberation (see Lahsen 2008).

Several of the most prominent advocates of this narrative that I interviewed in both Australia and the UK, for instance, expressed deep frustration at the slow rate of progress in policymaking on this issue. One said:

> And so we thought, 'Oh, gosh. Here goes another inquiry!' And I was actually gently quite sceptical, not because one can always do with more evidence, but how much evidence does one need? It's in bucketloads. (Interview with a British public health researcher, March 2012)

Another was even more emphatic:

> The evidence is in. It's not a debate. The evidence is there. (Interview with an Australian public health advocate, June 2011)

But other advocates of this narrative take the view that there is actually a distinct lack of evidence on obesity. One even confided:

> It is pretty much in my view an evidence-free area. There is virtually nothing proven to reduce or prevent obesity apart from famine and pestilence and they are the only evidence-based interventions you might consider. (Interview with an Australian researcher, July 2011)

Such differences can also lead to fractured claims around specific issues. The highest profile example involved the publication of Australia's future 'fat bomb' by the Baker Heart Research Institute in 2008. Based on findings from a survey of 3000 middle-aged people from across Australia, the report described obesity as a ticking 'time bomb' which necessitated urgent action. This invoked tremendous controversy, with some fellow adherents to the Structured Opportunity account strongly opposing this use and interpretation of evidence:

> Baker did this thing called the Fat Bomb—I thought that was outrageous. (Interview with an Australian public health advocate, June 2011)

Knowledge, Conflict, and Conciliation

Despite these considerably muddied waters, I want to be clear that there remains significant and obvious public contestation over knowledge claims around the issue of obesity in both Australia and the UK. The point is that the contestation is not clearly or solely limited to 'camps' or coalitions of actors who support particular narratives of the issue. Clashes in values, epistemological assumptions, disciplinary identities, and interest-based motivations generate discrepancies within narratives about obesity and overlaps across them.

What this all contributes to is a sense of paralysis. There is no agreement at any level of detail even among those who are seemingly on the same side. Naturally, this is a sense that can be reinforced by 'merchants of doubt' bankrolled by the food or medical industries, and I encountered some egregious examples in this research. In 2011, for instance, the Australian Food and Grocery Council (AFGC), the peak body for the processed food industry in Australia, funded a review of its advertising self-regulation regime. The findings, which the AFGC publicised widely, showed self-regulation had been a resounding success. Yet when a public health academic reproduced the study, she found that the AFGC had been disingenuous in its presentation of the data. This was, as some of my more outspoken interview participants suggested, straight from the 'Big Tobacco playbook'. More sombrely, a fellow adherent to the Facilitated Agency narrative noted with some discomfort:

> Kate Carnell [then CEO of the AFGC] got a very good run on that [initial study]. It was on the news. 'Oh well, that's pretty good evidence. Maybe that's okay then. Maybe it's not a problem.' But then someone looked at the study … I think that's really sloppy use of evidence from the Food and Grocery Council—very distorting. (Interview with an Australian health bureaucrat, July 2011)

But it would be wrong to attribute the uncertain sense of paralysis entirely to so-called 'merchants of doubt'. In fact, I suggest, it comes hand-in-hand with the hegemony of 'EBPM' that advocates buy into so deeply. Their overwhelming commitment to 'the evidence' means that competing knowledge claims about obesity can always be challenged and rejected. Indeed, contra widespread acceptance within mainstream public health scholarship about the 'cacophony' of having too many (loosely related) evidence-based solutions to obesity (see Lang and Rayner 2007), I have shown that virtually none are able to withstand scrutiny. All involve some leap of faith. Indeed, in line with the point made in the previous chapter about reflexivity, a number of public health experts (generally supporters of the Structured Opportunity or Social Dislocation accounts) across both countries confessed in interviews that, though in many ways an enabler of influence, their emphasis on 'EBPM' was inevitably an obstacle as well. One encapsulated this sense in a compelling reflection:

> There is a risk that we in the research area who are calling for more evidence-based policymaking may end up getting hoisted on our own petard: that it will be turned around and used against progress because there is not watertight proven evidence of effectiveness and cost-effectiveness. (Interview with an Australian public health expert, June 2011)

Conclusion

And so, far from convenient 'policy-based evidence', what I have revealed in this chapter is that contestation over the facts on obesity is complex and multifaceted. The politicisation thesis is as reductive and stylised as the depoliticisation thesis debunked in the previous chapter. There is no convenient alignment of facts in the service of a neater story. The widespread commitment to EBPM, and the range of commitments and beliefs that entails, mean that contestation over knowledge claims does not map neatly on to the divergent narratives outlined in Part 1. At times, in fact, the contestation within the coalitions that adhere to different narratives appears just as fierce as the contestation across diverging narratives.

The upshot, I have suggested, is a confusing and messy haze of knowledge claims. Virtually nothing about obesity is seen as settled, indisputable, unambiguous fact. Actors of all sorts, whether they broadly agree or not, remain at loggerheads over various aspects of the broader issue. And the result is a paralysis over detail that mitigates against the prospect of meaningful policy action at that level. All that is left is nebulous agreement at a high level of abstraction.

In the remaining chapter, and the conclusion, I want to focus on how knowledge claims make their way into policy work, how and why they inform policymaking, and to what effect. What I hope to show is that the contestation over knowledge claims outlined in this chapter leads to conciliation and compromise over ambiguous claims and categories, more acutely so in the Australian case where actors appear to feel more greatly constrained in their advocacy in elite and empowered institutional settings. The fierce contest over knowledge, I suggest, can actually obscure or mitigate against broader contestation over policy work and outcomes on this issue. Coupled with the dullening of emotion and exclusion of affected interests (as described in previous chapters), the effect is to manage the issue in Britain, and almost completely neutralise it in Australia.

References

Aphramor, L. (2009, May 9). All shapes and sizes. *The Guardian*. Retrieved January 15, 2013, from http://www.guardian.co.uk/commentisfree/2009/may/09/obesity-weight-health

Berg, C. (2008, January 6). Tackling obesity – Should the public pay?: The case against. *Sunday Age*. Retrieved January 15, 2013, from http://www.ipa.org.au/news/1523/tackling-obesity---should-the-public-pay-/category/9

Black, N. (2001). Evidence-based policy: Proceed with care. *British Medical Journal, 323*, 275–279.

Botterill, L., & Hindmoor, A. (2012). Turtles all the way down: Bounded rationality in an evidence-based age. *Policy Studies, 33*(5), 367–379.

Campbell, D. (2010, September 7). Call for more obesity surgery to cut benefits and NHS bills. *The Guardian*. Retrieved January 15, 2013, from http://www.guardian.co.uk/society/2010/sep/07/obesity-surgery-gastric-bypass

Colebatch, H. K. (2009). *Policy, 3rd ed.* Maidenhead, UK: Open University Press.

Cowell, L. (2010, March 18). The women who want to be obese. *The Guardian*. Retrieved January 15, 2013, from http://www.guardian.co.uk/lifeand-style/2010/mar/18/women-obese-donna-simpson-gainers

Fischer, F. (1995). *Evaluating public policy*. Chicago: Nelson-Hall Publishers.

Grube, D. (2012). Prime ministers and political narratives for policy change: Towards a heuristic. *Policy and Politics, 40*(4), 569–586.

Guilliatt, R. (2009, May 8). Off the scale. *The Australian*. Retrieved January 16, 2013, from http://www.theaustralian.com.au/news/features/off-the-scale/story-e6frg8h6-1225710631861

Hajer, M. A. (1995). *The politics of environmental discourse: Ecological modernization and the policy process*. Oxford: Clarendon Press.

Henry, J. (2008, April 20). "Obesity crusade" drives children to anorexia. *The Daily Telegraph*. Retrieved January 16, 2013, from http://www.telegraph.co.uk/news/uknews/1896136/Obesity-crusade-drives-children-to-anorexia.html

House of Representatives (HoR) Standing Committee on Health and Ageing. (2008, September 11). *Inquiry into obesity in Australia*. Sydney: Hansard, Australian Government.

Jolly, R. (2011). Marketing obesity? Junk food, advertising and kids. *Research Paper No. 9, 2010–11*. Australian Parliamentary Library, Canberra.

John, P. (1998). *Analysing public policy*. London: Continuum.

Jones, M. D., & McBeth, M. K. (2007). A narrative policy framework: Clear enough to be wrong? *Policy Studies Journal, 38*(2), 329–353.

Lahsen, M. (2008). Experiences of modernity in the greenhouse: A cultural analysis of a phyisicist "trio" supporting the backlash against global warming. *Global Environmental Change, 18*, 204–219.

Lang, T., & Rayner, G. (2007). Overcoming policy cacophony on obesity: An ecological public health framework for policymakers. Obesity Reviews, 8 (Suppl. 1), 165–181.

Lawrence, F. (2008, October 1). Britain on a plate. *The Guardian*. Retrieved January 17, 2013, from http://www.guardian.co.uk/lifeandstyle/2008/oct/01/foodanddrink.oliver

Lindblom, C. E. (1959). The science of "muddling through". *Public Administration Review, 19*(2), 79–88.

Marmot, M. G. (2004). Evidence-based policy or policy-based evidence? *British Medical Journal, 328*, 906–907.

Marmot, M. G. (2010, August 15). Ignorance is as big a killer as obesity. *The Observer*. Retrieved January 17, 2013, from http://www.guardian.co.uk/commentisfree/2010/aug/15/michael-marmot-health-wellbeing

O'Dea, J. A. (2010). Developing positive approaches to nutrition education and the prevention of child and adolescent obesity: First, do no harm. In J. A. O'Dea & M. E. Eriksen (Eds.), *Childhood obesity prevention—International research, controversies and interventions* (pp. 31–42). Oxford: Oxford University Press.

Oreskes, N., & Conway, E. M. (2010). *Merchants of doubt*. New York: Bloomsbury Press.

Parsons, W. (2002). From muddling through to muddling up – Evidence based policy making and the modernisation of British government. *Public Policy and Administration, 17*(3), 43–60.

Proietto, J. (2008, February 19). Surgery will do more than education to fix the obesity epidemic. *The Age*. Retrieved January 27, 2013, from http://www.theage.com.au/news/opinion/surgery-will-do-more-than-education-to-fix-the-obesity-epidemic/2008/02/18/1203190737640.html

Ryan, S. & Bita, N. (2009, January 9). Childhood obesity epidemic a myth, says research. *The Australian*. Retrieved January 17, 2013, from http://www.theaustralian.com.au/news/childhood-obesity-epidemic-a-myth/story-e6frg6n6-1111118515918

Sammut, J. (2008, April 33). Healthy lifestyles are taxing for everyone.

Sanderson, I. (2009). Intelligent policy making for a complex world: Pragmatism, evidence and learning. *Political Studies, 57*(4), 699–719.

Senate Standing Committee on Community Affairs. (2008, November 19). *Protecting children from junk food advertising (Broadcasting Amendment) Bill.* Canberra: Hansard, Australian Government.

Stone, D. A. (2002). *Policy paradox and political reason: The art of political decision making* (Rev. ed.). New York: W.W. Norton.

The Daily Mail. (2011, February 12). Future? What "f****** future?" The British estate where "healthy" life expectancy is just 58.8 years. *The Daily Mail*. Retrieved January 17, 2013, from http://www.dailymail.co.uk/news/article-1356247/Gurnos-Merthyr-Tydfil-The-British-estate-healthy-life-expectancy-just-58-8-years.html

The Sydney Morning Herald. (2009, January 14). Cut the excuses, not just the fat. *The Sydney Morning Herald*. Retrieved January 18, 2013, from http://www.smh.com.au/news/opinion/editorial/fit-the-crime-and-the-sentence/2009/01/13/1231608701607.html?page=2

Yanow, D. (1993). The communication of policy meaning: Implementation as interpretation and text. *Policy Sciences, 26*(1), 41–61.

Zimmet, P., & Jennings, G. (2008, February 22). Curbing the obesity epidemic. *The Age*. Retrieved January 18, 2013, from http://www.theage.com.au/news/opinion/curbing-the-obesity-epidemic/2008/02/21/1203467280758.html?page=fullpage

8

Transmitting Knowledge

Against the backdrop of limited and fractured public debates in Australia and the UK, advocates on this issue strive to impact on policy work. What I want to highlight here is that in doing so, they censor and moderate their knowledge claims considerably. They perform their preferred narrative with great strength, clarity, and specificity in the media (and even more so in their private interviews with me), but the overwhelming tendency—especially in the Australian case—is to mollify their account and leave copious 'wriggle room' for its interpretation as they encounter decision-making institutions. They do so largely out of a perception of what is appropriate, feasible, or likely to be adopted in policy work on this issue. As I will outline in depth, the fierce contestation over knowledge claims at a low level of specificity then gives way to muted conflict, indeed at times apparent agreement, at a high level of abstraction. And, in this sense, the backdrop described in Chaps. 5, 6, and 7 is important. With emotion and affect largely elided or sidelined from discussion, and rumbling conflict over seemingly every small detail, the reaction is to grasp for inoffensive, 'placebo' policies (see Gustafsson and Richardson 1979)—things like highly visible social marketing campaigns and kitchen-garden schemes. The politics underlying the issue of obesity

© The Editor(s) (if applicable) and The Author(s) 2016   **179**
J. Boswell, *The Real War on Obesity*,
DOI 10.1057/978-1-137-58252-2_8

becomes neutralised, albeit not to almost anyone's satisfaction dealt with. And the war on obesity largely peters out.

Much of what I have discussed so far in the analysis has applied equally to both countries but, as I will explain in greater depth, the trend I identify in this chapter is more pronounced—and its problematic ramifications more acute—in the Australian case than in the British one. I will use this chapter to outline how and why the seeming constraints on public advocacy apply more acutely in the Australian case, foreshadowing how this key discrepancy can help to unpack the drivers behind (and thus possible brakes to) the broader petering out of the political 'war on obesity'.

I build this argument over four important steps in this chapter. In the first, I look at the wide-ranging literature on issue containment in policy studies, particularly as it links to work on constructing issues and making knowledge claims. I do so to foreshadow how the findings I identify here challenge or extend these prevailing assumptions. In the second, I outline how actors (self-)censor and moderate their knowledge claims as they enter and approach formal institutions, illustrating how and why they do so. In the third, I highlight the effect of this censorship and moderation, in particular outlining how it leads to agreement or consensus around nebulous points of convergence, and can (in the Australian case especially) mitigate the prospect of renewed or sustained political debate. In the fourth, I conclude by returning to the lessons of this analysis for policy studies and public health work on issue and agenda management.

Knowledge, Advocacy, and Issue Containment

It is important to set the claims I want to make in this chapter against the prevailing orthodoxy in policy studies. Issue management or containment is a well-worn theme in this literature. A central interest of policy scholars has been on understanding how issues make it on to and off the public agenda. The findings I make here contribute to this work in two important, interrelated ways.

The first is to reiterate, as I alluded to in Chap. 4, that this literature tends to present issue management or containment solely as a deliberate (and even devious) strategy on the part of powerful institutional and corporate actors (see Thacher and Rein 2004). There is a burgeoning literature on the framing and priming of policy issues which presents political elites (as framers and primers) almost entirely as rational, utility-maximisers who exercise mastery over their own public discourse and its interpretation (see Iyengar 1991; Druckman and Nelson 2003; Druckman 2001). Even much of the more avowedly interpretive literature on narrative sees political elites as 'constructing' accounts in their effort to control the agenda (e.g. Grube 2012). What I hope to present here is an antidote to these accounts. My focus, inspired by much of the more thoughtful theorising on narrative in policy and politics (see Bevir and Rhodes 2003; Stone 2002; Hajer 2005), is, as I explained at the outset of the book, on narrative as live act, not dead text. In this sense, I build on a much more nuanced set of claims in this area about the situational, relational, polysemic environment in which elites attempt to influence public debate (see Finlayson 2007; Hajer 2009).

To be certain, I find compelling evidence of powerful actors (behind the dominant Facilitated Agency narrative) exploiting 'wriggle room' to block policy action and maintain the status quo. But the dynamic of issue containment, I suggest, is not entirely attributable to them, because the public agenda and the policy work that follows is not neatly under their control. It is as much a consequence of the actions and claims made by proponents of different, more critical narratives. The dynamic of issue containment in this case is not just a case of 'merchants of doubt' (see Oreskes and Conway 2010; Dryzek and Stevenson 2014; Moodie et al. 2013) obfuscating and blocking progress. Issue management or containment, I argue, is equally anticipated and (inadvertently) reinforced by critical actors in this debate as they (self-)censor and moderate their knowledge claims, more acutely so in Australia than in the UK.

The second contribution is that by far the most prominent work in this field tends to focus on agenda-setting and agenda management (Baumgartner and Jones 2009). Indeed, as I outlined in Chap. 3, the overwhelming tendency is to equate issue containment with the effort to constrict the scope of the issue in the agenda-setting phase. 'Getting obesity on the agenda' has, equally, been the primary focus in mainstream public health scholarship, too (see Brownell et al. 2009; Kersh 2009).

What my analysis reinforces, however, is that agenda-setting is only one aspect of policy work. There remains a very long march through the institutions of governance and policymaking through which a new issue on the agenda like obesity can become slowly eroded and mollified. I show how and why this occurs more acutely in the Australian case than in the British one. This comparison is instructive as discussion builds towards a conclusion focused on how the war on obesity might be rekindled and allowed to rumble on more effectively.

Censoring Knowledge Claims

I foreshadowed in Part 1, especially Chap. 3, a tendency towards self-censorship as actors approach empowered institutions of policymaking. I expound here on how adherents to more radical narratives on obesity either consciously or unconsciously opt not to advance these claims and instead reproduce more moderate narratives. I will explain this point, which happens to a much higher degree in Australia than in the UK, with reference to two stark and opposing examples.

The first example is an Australian food industry representative whom I interviewed in July 2011. In all of his public statements, and at the outset of our interview, this representative performed the Facilitated Agency narrative exclusively. He spoke at length about the complexity surrounding the issue, about the need to support individuals and families in making the right choices, and about the ongoing commitment of industry to be an active part of any solution to this problem. However, after we had built up something of a rapport, the tenor of his answers began to change. And, when asked about the absence of the Nanny State account from expert and decision-oriented sites of deliberation, he appeared to misunderstand my intention. He was not alone in doing so—many of those I spoke to assumed that in asking this line of question I was trying to advance this narrative personally, and some initially took great umbrage at the suggestion. Rather than feel offended, however, he opened up as if he felt safe to finally speak his mind:

[Experts talk about obesity as if it's a market failure.] It's not a market failure. It's a parenting responsibility failure. Yes, my kid nags me to buy the shiny packet of chips, lollies, soft drink, whatever, because of the way it's packaged. Absolutely. And there's a very easy answer to that, and that's 'no'. And she'll challenge it, and it'll be 'Sorry, darling, but the answer this time is the same as what it was last time. It's still no.' So I think that parents … what probably annoys me a little bit is that there seems to be all of these excuses, or all of these options for parents to abdicate their responsibility. It's … until the child is of working age and has their own disposable income then what goes in their mouth absolutely has to be the parents' responsibility, paring it back to its most basic issue. (Interview with an Australian food industry representative, July 2011)

The second example pertains to a public health researcher and advocate on the other side of the spectrum. This expert has a high public profile in Australia and is one of the best-known advocates of the Structured Opportunity narrative across all sites of deliberation. He is frequently in the media advocating for advertising restrictions and other key policy planks associated with the Structured Opportunity account. But in our interview—and in fact in a scholarly book that he has recently authored—this actor actually performed the Social Dislocation narrative. He explained:

Really deep in all this, really deep in terms of these determinants is our whole political and economic system is geared towards economic growth and consumption—a consumption-driven economic growth. Now I think countries like Bangladesh and Ethiopia desperately need some consumption-driven growth, but you get to a point where there's no added gains in human welfare however you measure it, and there's a huge amount of detriment in terms of overconsumption, and waste and carbon and obesity, all those things, they're all related to overconsumption. And it's this deep, deep belief that we have to have economic growth and we have to consume to make ourselves kind of happy and keep the economy ticking. That to me is the biggest issue. (Interview with an Australian public health researcher, June 2011)

In both cases, these actors appeared to be, wittingly or otherwise, self-censoring their advocacy. Rather than perform the Nanny State narrative, which is taboo in elite sites, or the Social Dislocation narrative, which is marginalised from debate in Australia almost entirely, both consistently reproduced more mainstream accounts in their public advocacy. They are, driven potentially by the demands placed on them in their public role, repressing the transmission of a narrative to which they subscribe.

The broader point I am trying to make through these two examples is not that these actors have been deceptive or disingenuous. Actors do not always align with a single narrative. They may also genuinely believe different things at different points of time. So, neither the performances they gave in our private interview nor those in their public advocacy should be seen as dishonest or misrepresentative of their views. In fact I found that almost without exception the backstage setting of the interview, in performative terms, elicited more radical performances than actors were willing to provide in the front-stage settings of public deliberation.

In response to my description of this phenomenon, one of my interview participants, and a close colleague of the public health advocate in question, explained the dynamic (to which he conformed somewhat, too) thus: 'How do you eat an elephant? You start with the first bite' (interview with a public health advocate, October 2012). His point was that advocates heavily engaged in policymaking discussions over a long period of time are conditioned to promote incremental but politically feasible measures, rather than campaign for major reform, regardless of their personal view.[1]

What is interesting is that while I did come across this general phenomenon in the UK, it was not nearly as prevalent as it seemed in Australia. One well-known proponent of the Social Dislocation narrative in the media, for instance, told me that he had tended to promote policies more in line with the Structured Opportunity narrative in expert deliberations and private discussions with decision-makers (interview with a British public health researcher, March 2012). Again, this can be read as reflecting a desire to influence policies that he perceived as feasible rather than to promote more radical alternatives which could easily be dismissed as unrealistic. But the important distinction here is that he did continue to perform the more radical Social Dislocation narrative across different sites of public deliberation, unlike his counterpart in Australia who reserved it solely for an academic audience. This comparative difference will be returned in the concluding discussion.

[1] This is consistent with what Carson (2008) finds in her reflections on the 2020 Summit, and the constraints placed on the event by the inclusion of mainly established advocates and experts.

Moderating Knowledge Claims

The other key factor is that the manner in which adherents to competing narratives on obesity advance knowledge claims in elite and empowered settings of debate serves to blunt the edge to the strongest critical accounts. In the media, the Structured Opportunity and (in Britain) Social Dislocation narratives, which challenge the status quo and demand far-reaching policy changes, are generally performed with great strength and clarity. Likewise, performances of these different accounts in a number of expert-dominated sites have been detailed, specific, and strong-worded in nature. Yet, as adherents to competing accounts have approached decision-oriented sites, their performances have typically generated far less clarity and strength.

This is especially apparent in relation to the Taskforce and the Foresight processes. These sites represented something akin to 'enclave deliberation' (Sunstein 2000)—these two advisory bodies comprised mainly like-minded experts who, when deliberating together in the relative absence of contradictory voices, pushed discussion in a more radical direction. Both featured a deliberately limited range of participants and points of view and, as a consequence, accommodated radical performances of the Structured Opportunity account (in particular) in their deliberations. For instance, a reading of the notes taken from roundtable consultations (with experts) of the Taskforce shows that most participants pushed strongly for major legislative and policy changes around the production, taxation, and marketing of food to cleanse the so-called 'toxic' environment. Accordingly, both the Taskforce and the Foresight processes have become closely associated with that account in their respective countries. But the outcomes of both these expert advisory processes, as they were fed into the government ministries under whose auspices they were run, have been greatly moderated.

The Taskforce is universally held in high regard by those who subscribe to the Structured Opportunity narrative in Australia. The process was, for those involved, 'gruelling', 'exhausting' but immensely satisfying. The outcomes of these deliberations, likewise, are collectively seen as a kind of manifesto. Yet a closer inspection shows that while the Taskforce process fostered radical performances of the Structured Opportunity narrative in its internal deliberations, its external contribution to the broader debate was far more constrained.

For a start, the public advocacy that surrounded the Taskforce was muted. One member of the Taskforce, for example, conceded that he felt limited in his public advocacy on the issue because of his links to the process. Voicing his opinions loudly in the press or elsewhere, he felt, could generate controversy and harm the legitimacy of the process. Moreover, despite the strong perception that the Taskforce's final report demands the sorts of policy actions that adherents to the Structured Opportunity narrative support, such as food labelling rules, marketing restrictions, and taxation changes, the document itself tells another tale. The wording of the report on all of these issues is much milder than that routinely used when this account is performed in the media. Instead of demanding regulations on junk food advertising, traffic light labelling, or a 'fat tax', the report merely suggests that the government 'restrict children's exposure to unhealthy food advertising', work collaboratively with industry to improve front-of-pack product labelling, and 'review the current system of taxes and subsidies' (National Preventative Health Taskforce 2009, pp. 15–18). The Taskforce report, according to one of the few advocates to speak out against it, represented a 'watering down' of the prevailing expert wisdom. On the television debate show *SBS Insight*, Boyd Swinburn claimed:

> Everything is being watered down. Even the existing documents that have been put together, the whole thing about reducing the intake of the unhealthy food and junk foods has been cleansed out of it. They talk about curbing inappropriate advertising to children during their children's hours—that is way too weak, way too watery.[2]

The same phenomenon was apparent in the UK with the Foresight process. Like the Taskforce, the Foresight process is closely associated with the Structured Opportunity narrative, with its report viewed as the clearest and most detailed account. Yet, as with the Australian Taskforce, the report was less radical than adherents to this narrative typically sug-

---

[2] See Boswell forthcoming for greater detail on the Taskforce and the moderation of claims.

gest. Indeed, the wording surrounding most recommendations is vague. Rather than demanding a raft of clear regulatory measures, the report suggests: redefining obesity as an environmental and social problem, not an individual one; taking a comprehensive, system-wide approach to the issue; developing long-term, sustained interventions; engaging with stakeholders in and out of government; and effectively monitoring changes (Foresight 2007, p. 14). None of these stated aims bear much resemblance to the strong rhetoric engaged in by proponents of the Structured Opportunity narrative in the internal deliberations.

Attaining 'Consensus'

These documents are symptomatic of a general tendency apparent in both cases for the actors in or closest to decision-oriented sites to advance knowledge claims that lack clarity and specificity. What results is an overlapping effort to converge around points of common ground. At first glance, in line with the orthodoxy in normative accounts of democracy, this sort of outcome would seem to be positive—as the lasting and legitimate culmination of democratic contestation over obesity. However, I will stress the dangers of attaining apparent 'consensus' at such a high level of abstraction.

The most striking example of such convergence occurs around the notion of 'complexity'. With the notable exception of advocates of the Nanny State account, everyone else in this debate acknowledges that obesity is a complex issue. A maxim repeated frequently on all sides is that 'there is no magic bullet', and that it is vital to acknowledge the complexity surrounding obesity. Indeed, 'complexity' came up in nearly all contributions to sites of deliberation, as well as every interview I held. In fact, I initially found myself tuning out in interviews when actors spoke about this point at length—hoping to move to another subject—only to realise later the significance of this universally agreed point.

This refrain to complexity is best illustrated in the 'obesity map' that was developed during the expert deliberations of the Foresight process in the UK. This map represents a systems analysis of all the contributing factors to obesity at both an individual and a societal level. Its intricate array of components and the overlapping connections between them visually represent the complexity of the issue—a point at the heart of not just most of the competing accounts on obesity, but in fact most performances of the respective accounts.

For example, Professor Louise Baur, a prominent advocate of the Structured Opportunity narrative in Australia, devoted a great deal of time and energy to conveying the complexity of obesity as a policy problem in her appearance at the HoR Inquiry. She explained to the MPs on the committee:

> Because there is such a mix of factors, the solution will not be simple. Many people would like to think there is one single thing we can do that would be enough to make a big difference, but that is very unlikely. These multiple causes are a real challenge for policymakers and also for science. (HoR Inquiry, September 11, 2008, p. 72)

Adherents to the Facilitated Agency narrative equally recognise the complexity of the problem. One explained to me in an interview:

> Nutrition is not rocket science; it's a whole lot harder. Because our relationship with food is so complex. There's cultural elements. There's safety elements. There's the sheer necessity of it—we all need it every day. There's cost elements. There's everything from the farm gate through to the most highly processed foods. (Interview with a senior Australian bureaucrat, June 2011)

Likewise, in response to an interview question about the impact of the change of government in the UK, an advocate of the Social Dislocation account played down the importance of the shift, explaining that he had been equally frustrated with the previous government's inability to grasp the complexity of the problem:

> But issues like obesity and overweight and the concomitant diseases that come with them ... They're about how we live ... [The participant outlines a long list of things rooted in the economic system such as transport, food supply, consumer culture and so on.] That complexity was completely lost on the Blair government. Completely lost. (Interview with a British researcher, May 2012)

Likewise, adherents to the Individual Intervention account make the same point, with one describing it as 'the most stigmatized and complex of chronic diseases' (McCallum 2008). And advocates behind the Moral Panic narrative make the same point, dismissing the claims of weight loss companies, pharmaceutical manufacturers, and surgeons who offer quick fixes:

> whatever the risks of a particular weight, the scientific evidence is clear: for the vast majority of people, there is no known safe way to obtain significant weight changes and maintain them in the long-term. (Aphramor 2009)

The corollary of complexity is a (near) universal commitment to a 'joined-up', 'coordinated', or 'whole of society' approach to dealing with obesity, and this language seeps unquestioningly into policy work in both Australia and the UK. However, bubbling tension lies beneath this superficial agreement around complexity and the need for coordinated or joined up governance. While in one sense the tropes provide useful points of consensus that brings adherents to different narratives together, in another they obscure ongoing disagreement over the precise nature of that complexity and, more importantly, over the implications of a 'coordinated approach' for policy decision-making on obesity-related regulations and initiatives.

Interpreting Consensus in Practice

Against the backdrop of fierce contestation over specific knowledge claims, actors reach for these nebulous points of conciliation—opening up considerable 'wriggle room' for the practical interpretation of apparent agreement and obscuring or masking key aspects of conflict in the process. I show that, in practice, this opens up space for powerful actors—especially the food lobby with its tremendous access and resources—to interpret 'wriggle room' associated with these vague policy commitments in ways that advance their interests.

In the UK, the Labour government, for instance, responded to the publication of the Foresight report by making obesity a major priority and setting up a specialist unit within the Cabinet Office. The rationale was that this unit would be able to work across the whole-of-government and provide the much needed 'coordinated response' that advocates of competing narratives had been calling out for in unison. Yet in practice the unit within the Cabinet Office, before it was disbanded by the incoming Coalition government, had achieved very little by way of tangible outcomes. The majority of policies that were pursued in the intervening time were ones which bore a striking similarity to those pursued in Australia at the same time, namely co-regulation of food marketing, voluntary labelling, and food reformulation (interview with a British food industry representative, March 2012; interview with a British researcher, March 2012). The fuzzy thinking behind the need for a 'coordinated approach' to this 'complex' problem had been whittled down—as far as many of my interview participants were concerned, because of the pressure brought to bear by the food industry and the inertia to cross-silo initiatives within the British bureaucracy—to a narrow and superficial understanding of what that might involve.

Again, however, this point is especially acute in Australia, and, returning to the discussion started in Chap. 6, is nowhere better demonstrated than in the rollout of the key policy plank of obesity prevention in Australia: the establishment of an arm's-length agency, the Australian National Preventive Health Agency (ANPHA). ANPHA has been trumpeted by some as a major policy achievement. Politicians, in particular, see it as evidence of their willingness to address obesity (and tobacco and alcohol control) in a proactive, coordinated manner (interview with an Australian politician, May 2011). Some others engaged in debate, including a few whose performances typically adhere to critical narratives on the issue, have expressed an equal degree of satisfaction with this outcome and optimism about ANPHA's role in policymaking around obesity (interview with an Australian NGO representative, June 2011). But many others who initially supported the move have begun to show signs of discontent. Some, reflecting on the 'ephemeral' nature of ANPHA and the way in which it has been brought into operation, see it as a 'toothless tiger' in practice (interview with an Australian clinician, June 2011). Others are concerned that its unsettled place in Australian health policymaking will make it little more than either a public relations tool for a government desperate to be seen to be doing something, or even worse, another channel through which the food lobby can wield its considerable influence. One prominent adherent to the Structured Opportunity narrative surmised in our interview:

> And my fear is that it's going to end up as a little bit of a weak follower of politicians' readiness to change. So in other words, it may well end up under the dynamic that there's enormous commercial lobbying, which influences the politicians enormously, which influences [ANPHA] enormously, so they will not be able to take a leadership role. And the fact that it's been based in Canberra means that it runs that risk a bit of kind of being captured within that political web of inactivity. (Interview with an Australian public health researcher, June 2011)

Others engaged in preventive health policymaking in Australia that I have spoken with in recent times have described ANPHA as effectively 'stillborn'. They have noted in particular that its profile has been kept intentionally low, that its activities have been limited to little more than funding health promotion programmes and a few academic workshops, and that it has been well and truly 'under the thumb' of the Department of Health, the leadership of which is notorious for its conservative approach towards, and desire to accumulate and retain control over, all aspects of health policymaking in Australia.[3]

My broader point is not that different interpretations of an ambiguous policy commitment are necessarily problematic. The literature on ambiguity in policy goals is long and unsettled one, with much work to suggest that such ambiguity is a persistent feature of policymaking. The long-standing orthodoxy has been that this characteristic is a problematic one—that it is indicative of an incomplete or flawed decision-making and design process, and that it is therefore something for policy analysts to work towards the eradication of (Mazmanian and Sabatier 1989). Others, in contrast, have recognised the ineliminability of goal ambiguity (Baier et al. 1986; Matland 1995; Kingdon 1995). Others still, with the emer-

---

[3] This concern was foreshadowed in an interview with an Australian health researcher in July 2011. It was then reinforced in private communication with an Australian health policy advocate in August 2012.

gence of interpretivism in policy studies, have actually begun to trumpet the value of goal ambiguity (see Hajer 1995; Stone 2002; Yanow 1993, 1996).[4] These authors point out that ambiguity is essential to the success of policies and programmes because it enables competing actors to 'buy in' to an outcome for different reasons. Ambiguity is thereby seen to buttress legitimacy and maintain progress in the governance of complex and contested issues.

However, the findings I make here align with recent interpretive scholarship in pointing equally to the dangers of ambiguity (see Smith and Kern 2009; Hudson 2006; Hupe et al. 2014; Bache et al. 2015; Zahariadis and Exadaktylos 2015). This emerging work reminds interpretive scholars that powerful actors can have tremendous influence over how ambiguous decisions are interpreted and transformed into formal decisions, and then especially over how such decisions are implemented. My findings on obesity show how the food lobby and health bureaucracy are well placed to exploit such advantages. In both cases, the food lobby have used their influence to steer policy in a way that favours their interests and goes against the wishes of many of those with whom they had seemingly reached agreement. In Australia in particular, they have done so in a way that neutralises the issue and forestalls ongoing debate on obesity—a point I expand on below.

Paralysing the Process

The process by which 'wriggle room' has developed around obesity in Australia has given the impression that the debate on this issue is over—that the contest of narratives has been won or at least a compromise between accounts forged. It is important to understand that obesity had been a very high-profile issue in Australia, and that its discussion in expert and decision-oriented sites actually served to heighten that exposure. Just

---

[4] There are clear affinities here with the work in science and technology studies on 'boundary objects'—a phenomenon whereby diverse actors coalesce around a particular idea or category such as complexity precisely because it is ambiguous and they are able to imbue it with their own preferred meaning. Lowy (1992) famously dubbed this 'the strength of loose concepts' (see also Star and Griesemer 1989 for a classic account).

prior to the 2020 Summit, for example, an open letter from four distinguished public health academics about the vital significance of obesity and the need to make this issue a key part of the forums' discussion was prominently placed in the *Sydney Morning Herald* (Caterson et al. 2008). Obesity also frequently made headlines during the HoR Inquiry. Indeed, it was around then that coverage of obesity reached a high point, with Melbourne broadsheet the *Age* running a memorable lead article entitled 'Nine million Australians are a ticking "fat bomb"'(Stark 2008b), which, in the wake of the 'fat bomb' report discussed earlier in the thesis, issued dire warnings about a wave of patients with complex, chronic diseases swamping the nation's health service. The article, and research report on which it was based, generated intensive discussion in the media. The Taskforce, too, generated headlines throughout its brief life, most notably when Kate Carnell gave up her post as CEO of the Australian General Practice Network—the advocacy body for general practitioners nationwide—to become the CEO of the Australian Food and Grocery Council, the peak body for the processed food industry, and continued as a member of the Taskforce. This instance of 'moving over to the dark side' (interview with a public health advocate, April 2011) stirred considerable controversy, resulting in greater media coverage and drawing more attention to the politicised nature of the issue (Stark 2008c).

However, once these innovative or one-time sites had run their course, the heat noticeably went out of the debate. One journalist I interviewed said that obesity was no longer a prominent news issue because there was 'nothing new about it' to discuss (interview with an Australian journalist, July 2011). This is not to suggest that there is no longer any coverage of the issue in the media, or that it is never discussed in Parliament, but obesity is clearly not the salient issue in the public sphere that it was 5 years ago.[5]

The issue here is that not only do key proponents of the dominant Facilitated Agency narrative in Australia such as food lobbyists have greater power to generate 'wriggle room' as decisions are reached and exploit this room as policies are implemented, they also have far greater power to

---

[5] This observation is based both on my personal assessment and on quantitative data that a colleague has generated through a content analysis of attention to obesity in the media and in Parliament in Australia (as yet unpublished).

impact on subsequent agenda-setting in the media or in Parliament. One very senior public health expert, for example, explained in an interview that he had been narrating Structured Opportunity behind the scenes intensively, informally lobbying a journalist he knows well to run a story on food industry interference in policy implementation. It was months before she finally aired a (one-off) report on Australian Broadcasting Corporation (ABC)'s *Lateline* (interview with an Australian public health researcher, July 2011). In contrast, a food industry representative—a key advocate of the Facilitated Agency account in Australia—boasted that, after a meeting in which she felt her concerns and ideas were not getting a fair hearing, she went back to her office and crafted a press release. The release suggested, tongue-in-cheek, that the government was planning to destroy an iconic Australian product by introducing restrictive regulations on food content. This prompted an immediate reaction, with the Prime Minister coming out publically promoting the brand within minutes (interview with an Australian food industry representative, May 2011). Likewise, prior to the 2007 federal election, for instance, the Labor Party had flirted with the idea of publicly performing the Regulatory Reform narrative. In particular, they had floated a proposal to crack down on advertising of junk food to children as part of the campaign. But a behind-the-scenes intervention by industry lobbyists convinced them to change their mind (McGarry 2007), and Labor's politicians have continued to adhere exclusively to the dominant Facilitated Agency narrative in their public statements ever since. Overall, in Australia, then, powerful actors have been able to draw on their economic and political resources to influence the political agenda and, ultimately, contribute to the neutralisation of the issue (at least for a time). But crucially, of course, their efforts must be seen to have been enabled and reinforced by the moderation of knowledge claims by proponents of critical narratives. It was a dynamic, performative, relational construction of 'wriggle room' in the first place.

The obesity debate in the UK exhibits many of the same features, save for one important difference. While there is an equally strong perception that government decisions and their execution have been influenced by powerful interests, and that successive governments have generally neutralised or watered down radical policies and ideas, there remains considerable public contestation over the substance of the issue and the perceived political injustices that have led to this juncture. In fact, obesity retained a similar salience throughout the period of analysis in the UK, or at least waxed and waned without the same pattern of decline apparent in Australia. The Responsibility Deals, for instance, provoked a resurgence of discontent among proponents of the critical Structured Opportunity and Individual Intervention accounts, resulting in screaming headlines such as: 'Fast food cave-in: Coalition strikes deal with Coca-Cola and McDonald's … but lets them regulate themselves' (*The Daily Mail* 2010) and 'Extent of corporate influence on health policy revealed: fast food and drink giants to help draft strategy' (Lawrence 2010). Indeed, the performances of leading politicians and government officials, and the policies and practices associated with them, have created something of a backlash, and the issue shot to near the top of the agenda again. One interview participant surmised:

> The way that the government has framed the debate I would say has been they very deliberately set out at the start that they wanted to take on sort of a collaborative approach and they wanted to involve industry. And I have to say in my experience the previous government did do that. So a lot of the previous government's policies, as with this government, were all voluntary initiatives. So the previous government did it, but this government really kind of set it out as if this is a great thing that we're doing and this is how we want to take it forward. It was a very public set down. I think that because of that there developed a really big backlash in the press and that actually made it a quite adversarial area to work in, which was exactly what they didn't want to happen. So the press very much took the stand of government isn't doing public health policy. It's allowing Coke and McDonald's and big chocolate bars to write the policy. That was very much the headlines. And that's been very much the rhetoric and the subsequent public health/obesity documents that have come out, they have been the type of headlines we've been getting. (Interview with a British food industry representative, March 2012)

Conclusion

The findings in this chapter, then, serve to challenge or at least augment the prevailing wisdom about issue containment and the battle over the public agenda. I have shown that the petering out of the obesity debate is not the evidence of the powerful food lobby's capacity to completely dominate the policy process, or control the public agenda. The very rise of obesity to the public agenda in Australia and the UK would seem to be a testament to their lack of mastery. Instead, I show how the complex interaction among proponents of different, more critical narratives across sites of democratic debate can generate wriggle room that powerful actors can capitalise on, though not create and control.

Here also I dwell on a major discrepancy between the two cases which sheds important light on these dynamics. I show how in Australia there is a heightened tendency for proponents of critical narratives to censor and modify their knowledge claims as they approach policymaking institutions, and to instead latch on to mutually agreeable but vague commitments surrounding complexity and the need for a coordinated approach. Having focused so intently on getting obesity on the agenda in the first place, these actors then have little capacity to effectively follow through on how ambiguous compromise is put into action, or rekindle broader debate about perceived failures or injustices in policy work. Powerful actors can better exploit this wriggle room. And the war on obesity is seen to be largely petering out. In the UK, in contrast, the greater reticence of critical actors to moderate their knowledge claims, coupled with an institutional architecture that better fosters and sustains ongoing critique, has meant less wriggle room for powerful actors to capitalise on as policy commitments are translated into action. Hence obesity as an issue has not been managed or contained to the same extent as in Australia, despite the similar backdrop of contestation over knowledge and marginalisation of emotion. The war on obesity rumbles on, albeit still in fits and starts.

The difference between the cases, in degree rather than in kind, informs a much more nuanced account of issue neutralisation than models of framing and agenda-setting predicated on assumptions about actor rationality. The findings here also re-problematise ambiguity in policymaking, not because it suggests an incomplete or flawed process of reaching decisions, but because it favours powerful interests in the messy, recursive process of translating vague agreement into action on the ground. It is the food lobby that can best exercise wriggle room, and they are able to wriggle away from unpalatable action more easily, and with less consequence, in Australia than in the UK. The reason, I argue, is that actors and governing institutions have been less equipped to track ambiguity through the policy process and enable scrutiny of its interpretation in practice.

Importantly for the conclusion that follows, these insights about the discrepancy between the cases can provide salient lessons for practical efforts to rekindle and sustain the political war on obesity. I turn my attention towards these conclusions now.

References

Aphramor, L. (2009, May 9). All shapes and sizes. *The Guardian*. Retrieved January 15, 2013, from http://www.guardian.co.uk/commentisfree/2009/may/09/obesity-weight-health

Bache, I., Reardon, L., Bartle, I., Flinders, M., & Marsden, G. (2015). Symbolic meta-policy: (Not) tackling climate change in the transport sector. *Political Studies, 63*(4), 830–851.

Baumgartner, F., & Jones, B. (2009). *Agendas and instability in American government* (2nd ed.). Chicago: University of Chicago.

Bevir, M., & Rhodes, R. A. W. (2003). *Interpreting British governance*. London: Routledge.

Boswell, J. (forthcoming). Deliberating downstream: Countering democratic distortions in the policy process. *Perspectives on Politics*.

Brownell, K. D., Schwartz, M. B., Puhl, R. M., Henderson, K. E., & Harris, J. L. (2009). The need for bold action to prevent adolescent obesity. *Journal of Adolescent Health, 45*, S8–S17.

Carson, L. (2008, April). 2020 Summit: Meetings in the foothills. *Australian Review of Public Affairs*. Retrieved January 29, 2013, from http://www.australianreview.net/digest/2008/04/carson.html

Caterson, I., Colagiuri, S., Nelson, M., & Zimmet, P. (2008, April 18). Government must tackle obesity, the tobacco of the modern age. *The Sydney Morning Herald*. Retrieved January 15, 2013, from http://www.smh.com.au/news/letters/government-must-tackle-obesity-the-tobacco-of-the-modern-age/2008/04/17/1208025372279.html

Druckman, J. N. (2001). On the limits of framing effects: Who can frame? *The Journal of Politics, 63*(4), 1041–1066.

Druckman, J. N., & Nelson, K. R. (2003). Framing and deliberation: How citizens' conversations limit elite influence. *American Journal of Political Science, 47*(4), 729–745.

Dryzek, J. S., & Stevenson, H. (2014). *Democratizing global climate governance*. Cambridge: Cambridge University Press.

Eaton Baier, V., March, J. G., & Saetren, H. (1986). Implementation and ambiguity. *Scandinavian Journal of Management Studies, 2*(3–4), 197–212.

Finlayson, A. (2007). From beliefs to arguments: Interpretive methodology and rhetorical political analysis. *British Journal of Politics and International Relations, 9*(4), 545–563.

Foresight. (2007). *Tackling obesities: Future choices—Project report (The Foresight Report)*. London: The Stationery Office. Retrieved January 18, 2013, from http://www.bis.gov.uk/assets/foresight/docs/obesity/17.pdf

Grube, D. (2012). Prime ministers and political narratives for policy change: Towards a heuristic. *Policy and Politics, 40*(4), 569–586.

Gustafsson, G., & Richardson, J. J. (1979). Concepts of rationality and the policy process. *European Journal of Political Research, 7*(4), 415–436.

Hajer, M. A. (1995). *The politics of environmental discourse: Ecological modernization and the policy process*. Oxford: Clarendon Press.

Hajer, M. A. (2005). Rebuilding ground zero: The politics of performance. *Planning Theory and Practice, 6*(4), 445–464.

Hajer, M. A. (2009). *Authoritative governance: Policymaking in the age of mediatization*. Oxford: Oxford University Press.

House of Representatives (HoR) Standing Committee on Health and Ageing. (2008, September 11). *Inquiry into obesity in Australia*. Sydney: Hansard, Australian Government.

Hudson, B. (2006). User outcomes and children's services reform. *Social Policy and Society, 5*, 227–236.

Hupe, P., Nangia, M., & Hill, M. (2014). Studying implementation beyond deficit analysis: Reconsidering the top-down view. *Public Policy and Administration, 29*, 145–163.

Kersh, R. (2009). The politics of obesity: A current assessment and look ahead. *Milbank Quarterly, 87*(1), 295–316.

Kingdon, J. W. (1995). *Agendas, alternatives and public policies*. London: Longman.

Lawrence, F. (2010, December 9). Extent of corporate influence on health policy revealed: Fast food and drink giants to help draft strategy. *The Guardian*. Retrieved January 17, 2013, from http://www.guardian.co.uk/politics/2010/dec/09/health-policy-extent-corporate-influence

Lowy, I. (1992). 'The strength of loose concepts—Boundary concepts, federated experimental strategies and disciplinary growth: The case of immunology. *History of Science, 30*, 371–396.

Matland, R. E. (1995). Synthesizing the implementation literature: The ambiguity-conflict model of policy implementation. *Journal of Public Administration Research and Theory, 5*, 145–174.

Mazmanian, D. A., & Sabatier, P. A. (1989). *Implementation and public policy.* Washington, DC: University Press of America.

McCallum, Z. (2008, April 27). Far too much to lose. *The Sunday Age.* Retrieved January 17, 2013, from http://www.theage.com.au/news/opinion/far-too-much-to-lose/2008/04/26/1208743319461.html

McGarry, A. (2007, November 6). Pollies gutless on obesity: Health guru. *The Australian.* Retrieved January 17, 2013, from http://www.theaustralian.com.au/news/health-science/pollies-gutless-on-obesity-guru/story-e6frg8y6-1111114810006

Moodie, R., Stuckler, D., Monteiro, C., Sheron, N., Neal, B., Thamarangsi, T., et al. (2013). Profits and pandemics: Prevention of harmful effects of tobacco, alcohol, and ultraprocessed food and drink industries. *Lancet, 381*, 670–679.

Oreskes, N., & Conway, E. M. (2010). *Merchants of doubt.* New York: Bloomsbury Press.

Preventative Health Taskforce. (2009). *Australia: The healthiest country by 2020.* Australian Government, Department of Health and Ageing, Canberra. Retrieved January 18, 2013, from http://www.preventativehealth.org.au/internet/preventativehealth/publishing.nsf/Content/AEC223A781D64FF0CA2575FD00075DD0/$File/nphs-overview.pdf

Smith, A., & Kern, F. (2009). The transitions storyline in Dutch environmental policy. *Environmental Politics, 18*(1), 78–98.

Star, S. L., & Griesemer, J. R. (1989). Institutional ecology, "translations" and boundary objects: Amateurs and professionals in Berkeley's museum of vertebrate zoology, 1907–39. *Social Studies of Science, 19*(3), 387–420.

Stark, J. (2008b, June 20). Nine million Australians are a ticking "fat bomb". *The Age.* Retrieved January 17, 2013, from http://www.theage.com.au/national/nine-million-australians-are-a-ticking-fat-bomb-20080619-2tjv.html

Stark, J. (2008c, November 23). Taskforce tainted, say health groups. *The Sunday Age.* Retrieved January 17, 2013, from http://www.theage.com.au/national/taskforce-tainted-say-health-groups-20081122-6eis.html

Stone, D. A. (2002). *Policy paradox and political reason: The art of political decision making* (Rev. ed.). New York: W.W. Norton.

Sunstein, C. R. (2000). 'Deliberative trouble?: why groups go to extremes'. *Yale Law Journal, 110*, 71–119.

Thacher, D. & Rein, M. (2004). Managing value conflict in public policy. *Governance, 17,* 457–486.

The Daily Mail. (2010, December 1). Fast food cave-in: Coalition strikes deal with Coca-Cola and McDonald's … but lets them regulate themselves. *The Daily Mail.* Retrieved January 18, 2013, from http://www.dailymail.co.uk/news/article-1334475/Coalition-Coca-Cola-McDonalds-strike-deal-fight-obesity.html

Yanow, D. (1993). The communication of policy meaning: Implementation as interpretation and text. *Policy Sciences, 26*(1), 41–61.

Yanow, D. (1996). *How does a policy mean?: Interpreting policy and organizational actions.* Washington, DC: Georgetown University Press.

Zahariadis, N., & Exadaktylos, T. (2015). Policies that succeed and programs that fail: Ambiguity, conflict, and crisis in Greek higher education. *Policy Studies Journal, 44*(1), 1–129. doi:10.1111/psj.12129.

9

Conclusion

In one interview with a prominent public health representative, the participant concluded our discussion by describing to me the first ever episode of *The Hollowmen*. This was a popular (among political insiders) political satire set in the fictional Central Policy Unit (CPU) in Canberra, and its first episode had screened a couple of years prior. The show she was referring to charts the CPU's efforts to follow through on the Prime Minister's strong (and off-the-cuff) commitment to tackling obesity. The team begins with a concrete, six-point plan of action based on seemingly the best available advice. But, as the food industry weighs in, and the implications for the rest of government become clear—the Sports Minister, for example, is furious at the prospect of lost sponsorship revenue—they are left to extricate themselves from meaningful action and save face with a few visible but tokenistic programmes. The six-point plan is reduced to two shaky pillars: 'a code of conduct' for the food industry and 'an awareness campaign' for the public. The episode ends with a glimpse of the Prime Minister in a carrot costume on his way to the launch of this campaign.

Though screened in 2008, this account would prove, as my analysis has laid bare, frighteningly prescient. Substitute the carrot costume for an

J. Boswell, *The Real War on Obesity*,
DOI 10.1057/978-1-137-58252-2_9

animated balloon man—the social marketing campaign centred around 'Eric the Swapper', a blue balloon man in need of gentle deflating—and the story is much the same. But this is not just a case of life imitating art. The interview participant who drew my attention to the episode had been the key advisor to the show's writer. Its cynical prediction is a product of her own fatalism. She reflected:

> I said to someone that we finally reached the end of that episode with the blue man … Thank God that's over. The relief. I was just waiting for it to finish. My life has just played out. The Hollowmen did it in 40 minutes. It took me 4 years. (Interview with an Australian public health advocate, June 2011)

This anecdote provides a telling insight into the frustrations that actors themselves feel with the complex politics of obesity (see Boswell and Corbett 2015b). What I have attempted to show in this analysis, however, is that this outcome is not entirely attributable to political neutralisation and food industry obfuscation (as the quoted participant would suggest). The dynamics of the famed 'issue attention cycle' (Downs 1972), as revealed here, involve a complex interplay of knowledge, advocacy, and power into which advocates for change themselves contribute significantly.[1] I will briefly recap the argument to hammer this point home.

In Part 1 of the book, I demonstrated that the debate on obesity is much more than a 'war' between interests in the food industry and those in public health, certainly not one fought along a clear ideological divide between structure and agency, or amid colliding efforts to 'politicise' or 'depoliticise' the issue. In Chap. 2, I showcased the significant overlaps in the way this apparent 'food fight' between two clear camps plays out in practice. I show that the primary narratives on obesity in Australia and the UK—the dominant Facilitated Agency account and its primary counter, Structured Opportunity—converge and overlap at significant points. In Chap. 3, I outlined two expert-led narratives that at times not only overlap but also diverge significantly from these primary accounts—one the

---

[1] There are important parallels to my findings in the complex connections between discursive politics and issue and agenda management in the excellent recent analysis by Griggs and Howarth (2013) of the ongoing debate about aviation policy in the UK.

Individual Intervention narrative, the other the Social Dislocation narrative. These accounts do not just foreshadow the uncertainty over scientific evidence on this issue, they highlight that contestation among policy actors can be as much over the appropriate scope of the issue as about the type or nature of intervention required. In Chap. 4, I complicated the picture further, highlighting two radical narratives that challenge the very existence of this problem—one, an old and familiar Nanny State account whose proponents acerbically challenge the classification of obesity as a public (rather than private) concern, and the other, an emergent critical account of Moral Panic that challenges the very problematisation of obesity at all. Along the way, Part 1 speaks to important debates in policy studies about the role and nature of narrative in political debate, and its relationship to battles over the scope of policy issues or their place on the public agenda. The analysis starts to reveal that the knowledge politics of obesity is considerably more nuanced and complex than existing work on the social construction of the issue tends to countenance.

Using this background as the basis of Part 2 of the book, I have richly depicted the stalled 'war on obesity' encapsulated in *The Hollowmen* episode. However, unlike this stylised representation (one undertaken not just for humorous effect), I have presented it less as the successful efforts of all-powerful and shadowy elites to control debate and more as the product of a complex set of dynamics as adherents to these different narratives represent, claim, contest, and transmit knowledge across debate. In Chap. 5, I argued that the marginalisation of obese voices blunts the emotional edge to this issue and, inadvertently, reinforces old stigmas about the capacity and deservingness of obese individuals. In Chap. 6, I showed that the widespread deference to scientific evidence not only enables mutual (and somewhat inclusive) engagement and contestation on this issue, but also reinforces rational norms that further sideline emotion. I expanded on this point in Chap. 7, showing how the emphasis on evidence within a context of ongoing uncertainty generates a haze of confusing and contradictory knowledge claims, mitigating the prospect of action on specific policy measures. In Chap. 8, I built on this by showing how expert representatives adapt and soften their knowledge claims as they approach decision-making institutions, pursuing nebulous points of agreement at a high level of abstraction, which are almost inevitably steered in the interests of powerful actors and away from anything that challenges the status quo.

So, powerful actors like the food lobby have not been able to completely control the agenda. What they have been better able to do is exploit the resultant 'wriggle room' as debate about obesity is turned into policy action. The problem I want to emphasise here is not that such dynamics engender a watery or tokenistic policy response. With such palpable uncertainty, complexity, and polarisation surrounding the issue, it is hard to imagine any other outcome. Instead, the key danger is that in the generation of this stalemate, more acutely so in the Australian case where actors have felt more constrained in what they can advocate for, there is removed impetus for further contestation and debate. The real war on obesity—the political contest over its nature and meaning in policy terms—risks petering out.

As such, this conclusion focuses on the lessons that can be gleaned from this analysis in order to reignite policy debate and ensure greater attention and scrutiny for this issue. The insights emerge both from analysis of the slight discrepancies between the cases, drawing on key features which might explain Britain's slightly more active and sustained political debate, and from an account of the common drawbacks and pathologies in both cases. They are designed to more broadly inform the policy studies literature, pointing to new governing practices and institutions that might speak to problems and pathologies in cognate policy fields. However, they may be of equal value to (critical) public health scholars, helping them to understand ways in which their advocacy efforts may be more fruitfully directed in order to better sustain the political war on obesity.

From Expert Representation to Affective Embodiment

Chapter 5 explored the most lasting, curious, and manifestly problematic impression of the obesity debates in Australia and the UK—that almost none of the credible advocates of any of the competing narratives outlined in Part 1 is themselves obese. Most of those engaged in debate are vehement about their empathy for the plight of obese individuals, and they claim to represent their interests, as Role Models, Carers, or Nannies. Yet, as I show, there are limitations to this form of *discursive representation*. Discursive affinity alone is insufficient. The symbolic domain of democratic politics contains much more than mere language. And so, I show, expert or elite delegates may be able to rehearse competing narratives effectively, but they cannot necessarily represent them. The empathetic impulse underlying these claims can be undermined by their performative implications. The absence of obese actors from expert or decision-making institutions in both countries inadvertently reinforces the old stigma about obesity as a deviant, private condition. It undercuts the avowed message of empathy and professed claims for education, treatment, or consumer protection. This very invisibility, of course, resonates with one of the key claims for 'the politics of presence'.

Yet, to be clear, in this case evidence supporting the primary claim of *descriptive representation*—that it enables the representation of substantive interests that would not otherwise have voice—is not so clear-cut. Proponents of all the competing narratives are more than willing to couch their claims in terms of personal, local, embedded knowledge on obesity. Role Models, of course, can share their own personal stories. Carers can talk about the patients with whom they feel such strong bonds. And even Nannies are typically quick to frame their concerns in relation to the everyday experience of the 'victims' they seek to protect.

It is not *substance* missing so much, then, as *affect*. Affect is in this sense the physical rendering of human feelings in political contestation (Thompson and Hoggett 2012). The discursive—the narrative texts—captures much of value and interest for policy and politics scholars but, of course, meaning is conveyed in other subtle and important ways in policy debate. Facial expressions, pitch and tone, body language, objects, interactions—these are all ways of communicating that engage the affective rather than (or as well as) the discursive. Scholars are beginning to disentangle the important influence of the affective in political communication, revealing how it can serve to reinforce but also undermine the discursive in policy debate. Indeed, this represents one of the most exciting, burgeoning fields in interpretive political science and policy studies (see Newman 2012).

There is strong reason to believe that affective aspects of communication are especially important in the context of obesity. Obesity is, after all, a condition that is itself unmistakably and poignantly *embodied* (see Warin et al. 2008; Kline 2015). Of course, obesity is not alone in being a condition that actors embody. Race, gender, disability, and so on, are all embodied as well. So when debate centres on gender equality in the labour market, indigenous land rights, or disability benefits, those are all issues in which actors can unmistakably embody the concern at stake. But obesity is different because it remains imbued with moral stigma—while you are not responsible for your gender, ethnicity, or disability, and you cannot do anything about it, the background message remains that you are responsible for your weight, and that you can do something about it (Gard and Wright 2008; Lupton 2013). To be clear, many policy issues or problems centre around problematic 'targets' who exhibit deviant behaviour. Indeed, some of the greatest challenges facing policymakers are a consequence of predominant lifestyle choices (and the difficulties associated with shifting those choices). But individuals do not necessarily exhibit the hallmarks of a smoker, a drinker, or a drug addict, let alone an SUV driver or a reluctant recycler. Obesity is physically embodied at all times. So it is the combination of these two factors that makes obesity such a difficult case, and one where the lack of affective embodiment is such an important deficit in the democratic contestation of this issue.

My analysis shows how competing narratives on obesity, as they are performed across sites, lose some of their critical edge and emotive appeal. I contend that the deference to elite and expert delegates contributes to this dynamic. As I showed in Chap. 5, some of the most moving experiences for politicians engaged in the *Weighing it Up Inquiry* in Australia were when they were confronted with the emotion of obesity viscerally— on being confronted with graphic physical representation of pain and discomfort, on site visits to clinics and community centres, in informal discussions with obese individuals and their loved ones. More regular engagement with such affective embodiment would make it much harder to allow the stalemate in policy debate to continue. It would help keep the real war on obesity rumbling on.

Public health scholars who seek to achieve regulatory change would also do well to take heed of the importance of such symbolism. My analysis shows that they are widely perceived as elitist 'zealots'; they are seen as a chorus of Nannies, whose calculated distance leaves them out of touch with ordinary people, and who seek to regulate and control the lifestyles of these people they do not know (and implicitly, do not approve of). They may see the food lobby, or the socio-economic order, as the enemy. But in calling for food taxes or product reformulation, they risk being perceived as 'micro fascists' (as in Rail et al. 2010), imposing their will on ordinary people and denying them simple pleasures in their daily life.

For these actors, then, it seems that opening obesity back up to genuine, intense, and prolonged public debate will require forming a looser coalition with a greater diversity of actors, including civil society actors and engaged citizens who feel passionate about this issue. Above all, this will mean sharing the stage with obese individuals themselves, whose voice has hitherto been marginalised or crowded out of policy discussions. There is of course a risk that in making the coalition more diffuse they further dilute the purity of the account. But it seems likely that what is lost in discursive affinity can be made up for in the performative appeal of having the most affected public actively engaged. As such, I suggest that public health actors hoping to influence policymaking on obesity would do much better to stand alongside, rather than in the way of or on behalf of, the most affected public that they claim to represent.

From Emotional Evidence to Evidence on Emotions

Chapter 6 explored the knowledge claims made by proponents of competing narratives on obesity, focusing especially on the universal 'fetish' for evidence in relation to this issue in both cases. At first glance this would appear to be dismal news for the democratic qualities of policy debate on obesity, underpinning precisely the sort of technocratic rationality that has long worried critical policy scholars. Yet I have argued that the universal commitment is not all bad. I show that the evidence on obesity is, to some extent, democratised, with actors of all sorts capable of drawing on scientific evidence to support their claims. Moreover, I show that a commitment to EBPM does not entail an unreflective negation of other sources of knowledge. My findings suggest that actors are highly reflexive about the limitations of EBPM and the need to draw together evidence with other important sources of knowledge, such as professional practice, personal experience, ethical claims, and cultural wisdom.

Indeed, not only is the fetish for evidence not all bad, it is actually in one important way quite beneficial for democratic governance. The focus on evidence provides a basis for what normative theorists of democracy call reciprocity (see Gutmann and Thompson 1996)—a commitment to couching claims in a manner that all the actors engaged in debate can accept (even if they contest the interpretation).[2] And reciprocity is the essential ingredient in legitimacy, enabling rival actors to remain stoically committed to the process in the face of the endless frustration associated with complex policy work. Adherents to these competing narratives keep up the good fight in the hopes that 'the truth will out', and that the evidence which supports their account of obesity will become overwhelmingly compelling. What emerges is far from the depoliticised reach for technocratic rationality that so concerns critics of EBPM (see Boswell 2014 for more).

However, my analysis does uncover a more subtly problematic consequence of the fetish for evidence in these debates. That is, related to the point above, the sidelining of the emotional experience of obesity. To be very clear, my claim is not that the debate is dispassionate. There is a tendency in the aforementioned 'affective turn' in politics and policy studies (see Thompson and Hoggett 2012) to see emotions as the preserve of marginalised or un-mobilised publics and to contrast that with the apparently robotic or cynical rationality of political elites. But my analysis, and in particular my interviews with key actors, has shone light on something that is fairly obvious if not always acknowledged: elites have feelings, too.

---

[2] It is worth noting that there are affinities between my appeal to reciprocity and the emphasis on 'boundary work' deployed by policy scholars like Hoppe (2005, 2013) and Korinek and Veit (2015). Boundary work in this sense draws on insights from science and technology studies, and in particular insights into practices of regulatory governance where the divergent discourses or 'sacred stories' of scientists, professionals, and policymakers intersect (see Jasanoff 1990, 1996). Evidence is, likewise, a crucial part of what enables boundary work to actually work in practice. I prefer the term *reciprocity* here because it is avowedly normative and points to underappreciated democratic benefits associated with the supposedly technocratic pursuit of EBPM (see Boswell 2014 for much more on this).

Adherents on all sides are often very emotional about the issue—deeply concerned or sometimes enthusiastic, deeply frustrated or sometimes energised, deeply resigned or sometimes hopeful. What is more, in more open, public settings, they typically go out of their way to imbue their avowedly evidence-based accounts with emotion: they deliver *emotional evidence*. Yet as actors reproduce these accounts in or near empowered sites of policy decision-making, as I reveal in Chap. 8 especially, this emotional edge becomes blunted in the search for a 'realistic' compromise. This muting of emotion makes it much easier for watery, tokenistic compromise to pass with little fanfare or scrutiny, and for the war on obesity to peter out.

To mitigate this tendency—so apparent in the obesity cases but something that also resonates with other deeply emotional issues—I call here not for an end to emotional evidence, but for augmentation with greater *evidence on emotions*. Providing more coherent, persuasive evidence on the emotional impact for individuals can help to legitimate and sustain the emotional edge to this issue. Social scientists, especially scholars of an interpretive or critical orientation, are only now beginning to unpack the emotions associated with obesity and the various campaigns/treatments that follow from it (see Banwell et al. 2013; Orsini 2015). Unveiling, packaging, and promoting this knowledge under the banner of social science can give voice to the marginalised in a way that works with, rather than against or in subordination to, the 'evidence-based' norms of prevailing debate.

Sceptics will be quick to note that the sort of evidence I have in mind—largely qualitative, anecdotal—sits low on the 'hierarchy of evidence' in health policymaking, and that it thus seems unlikely to exercise much influence on debate (see Milewa and Barry 2005). Yet, as I showed in Chap. 6, there is a reflexive understanding among actors engaged in this debate that this hierarchy is not a neat fit for such a complex issue, and that there is appetite for considerably more fluidity and flexibility in piecing together compelling evidence for policy action. Evidence on emotions can be a crucial part of any such mix, and one that is uniquely likely to *affect* policymakers (Orsini and Scala 2006). It can legitimate, and ensure continued high-profile discussion of, the affective experience of obesity to which almost everyone can intimately relate. At the very least, it seems that more reference to evidence on emotions would be likely to sustain impetus for continued debate and contestation on complex and contested issues like obesity.

This message is also important for public health scholars with an interest in rekindling the war on obesity. Reference to scientific evidence remains, of course, the particular trump card of these experts, and it hardly seems profitable for them to forego such an advantage by refraining from discussing the evidence. But my analysis shows just how subject to divergent interpretation the evidence can be, and therefore how limiting, and ultimately self-defeating, it can be for advocates to rest their claims *solely* in these terms, especially when the prevailing evidence remains subject to refutation. My analysis reveals the importance of emotional appeals in attracting attention, persuading influential actors, and gaining lasting influence in policy work. As such, drawing on the reflections of some of the most experienced public health activists and advocates involved, I argue that these actors would do well not to downplay or marginalise the emotional aspect of this issue, nor to look down on softer social science techniques for developing and understanding the lived experience of obesity. Evidence on these emotions can be a key part of the mix in trying to influence change.

Between Conflict and Conciliation

Chapter 7 sheds light on how knowledge on obesity is contested across debate. Contra simplistic assertions about 'policy-based evidence' and the cynical manipulation of science, I show that actors do not just use the 'facts' in service of a neater account. I outline a hazy, shifting map of knowledge claims. I find an overwhelming sense of paralysis as actors who so strongly advocate for EBPM become 'hoisted on their own petard'. These insights take on particular import when set against the findings in Chap. 8, which show how actors mute and moderate their claims as they move across sites of debate. In both cases, the sense of paralysis surrounding any discrete, concrete policy proposal begets a shared commitment to compromise at a higher level of abstraction. Competing narratives intersect around ambiguous claims (such as complexity) and goals (such as a whole-of-society response), which powerful actors in the food lobby especially are able to steer in their interests as they draw on their resources to better 'stay' with the issue through processes of implementation. Here I return to an important discrepancy between the two cases, albeit one better understood as a difference of degree or intensity rather than kind.

In Australia, the drive for conciliation within elite and empowered sites of decision-making does not just result in policy 'wriggle room'; it seems to actively undercut impetus for further contestation. Recall that back in Part 1, in Chaps. 3 and 4, I showed how adherent to radical narratives on obesity felt conditioned by accepted interpretations of feasibility, such that they refrained from performing accounts (at either end of the spectrum) altogether. Equally, this fear of being perceived as unreasonable, perhaps driven by the famously pragmatic tradition (or some might say myth) which characterises and conditions Australian policymaking (see Wanna and Weller 2003), seems to drive many to suppress or control their frustration or resentment at policy inaction. Experts and NGOs, who are relative newcomers to governance networks and who thus have a precarious place within them, appear desperate not to risk their hard-won inside influence by publicly expressing disapproval (see Boswell and Corbett 2015b for more on this). Instructive here is consideration of an important exception, Public Health Association of Australia (PHAA) CEO, Michael Moore.[3] Moore explained how he was willing to risk his network insider status by publicly criticising government, largely because he recognised that this status was not really at risk. He had the relationships and trust with other actors to allow him to do that—none stronger or more long-running than with notorious food lobbyist Kate Carnell. He revealed how he was willing to publicly lock horns with Carnell over public health on the back of years of similar experience serving as an independent Health Minister in her Liberal ACT government:

> I've had this ongoing relationship with Kate for 20 years, where actually we've always both understood that conflict is part of getting our message through. And because we actually understand that, sometimes it's actually quite useful. And in fact we've had in the past within the political sphere, when I was a Minister in her government but I was opposing something— because I was an independent minister there were things that I opposed the

---

[3] I thank Michael for allowing me to quote him by name, or else his identity would not be obvious and I would not be able to use this remarkable insight.

government on where I wasn't held by ministerial solidarity and we would actually discuss beforehand the way this sort of conflict was going to go. Generally it went the way we had expected it to. So as far as the general public was concerned there we were having a very significant debate—and we did, we had a genuine difference of opinion—but we were also—we may have looked like we were cross at each other or something but in fact it was quite orchestrated. (Interview with Michael Moore, April 2011)

A handful of others shared Moore's conviction but the bulk, in action more so than personal reflection, seemed desperate not to 'rock the boat'. The result has been intense, multifaceted conflict giving way to watery, tokenistic compromise. And the war on obesity in Australia risks petering out.

In Britain, in contrast, civil society remains, in the words of one interview participant, 'articulate and confident'. There is greater willingness to give voice to radical narratives. There is also greater willingness among network insiders to be openly critical. There has been, for instance, a coordinated outcry and large-scale walkout associated with the Coalition government's Public Health Responsibility Deals, under the perception these governance mechanisms would be dominated by industry interests. Australia's Food and Health Dialogue, in contrast, carried on away from the headlines despite grave misgivings (of a similar nature) among many actors. Indeed, British interview participants were very matter-of-fact that they saw it as their duty to pursue dual insider and outsider advocacy strategies. The result is that conflict keeps bubbling away to a greater degree, and the war on obesity rumbles on, albeit still in fits and starts.

These insights have significant purchase for ongoing debates about the mix of contestation and conciliation in democratic governance. The recent resurgence of deliberative approaches to democratic policymaking—approaches that promote consensual conciliation rather than the older tradition of adversarial contest—has come in for increasing criticism for its capacity to constrict or control debate and to pave the way for the marginalisation of vulnerable actors (see Sanders 1997; Blaug 2002). There is increasing recognition, even among avowed deliberative democrats, that adversarial advocacy remains essential in doses (Mansbridge et al. 2010; Hendriks 2011). One of the most interesting recent reflections on this point is the work of Stefan Rummens (2011) on 'democratic stages' in systems of representation in contemporary liberal democracies. He emphasises the importance of democratic venues that encourage the active performance of opposition to legislative and administrative action. Recognising the ineliminability of conflict over complex and contentious issues, he astutely sees the ongoing, dynamic forms of representation these stages enable as working to publicise the contingent or unsatisfactory nature of deliberative outcomes. Though Rummens remains focused on the established set pieces enacted in existing institutional architectures, the case work at hand—and the differences between them—extends these insights through the policy process. Here, as 'wriggle room' is negotiated, and vague commitment is turned into action, there appear many more institutional opportunities for sustaining democratic contestation along with the compromise required in actually getting things done—and it is to this extension of such opportunities through the policy process that I turn my attention in the next section.

First, though, it is important to briefly consider the implications of this insight for a public health audience. Public health activists could also be savvier about the ways in which they engage with government actors and especially 'the enemy' in the food industry. Though there is a strong perception of a polarised obesity debate, in fact what this analysis reveals is that little scrutinised moves towards conciliation in policy work behind closed doors represent a bigger danger, as conflict among experts about the fine detail displaces conflict between political actors about broad matters of policy direction and principle. Once more, drawing on the reflections of the activists involved, and from the stronger performance of British advocates on this dimension, my analysis shows that public health experts ought to be more assertive about their place at the policymaking table and less afraid to publicise their concerns about the fairness of opaque stakeholder deliberations. They can thereby sharpen the conflict that the ambiguous compromises reached through these venues tend to elide and mask.

Between Input and Output

The petering out of debate that I describe in Part 2 also points to another important implication—and that is, in line with some of the most recent work on discursive politics, to focus analytical (and practical) efforts on governing *throughput* just as much as is typically reserved for *input*. This notion draws on the terminology employed by Vivian Schmidt (2013)—though originally indebted to the seminal work of David Easton (1965)—to capture the components of democratic governance. *Input*, in this sense, is tightly associated with agenda-setting and the effort to prime and frame issues for legislative attention and decision. *Output* is the administration of that given decision, in the form of policies and programmes. In between the two is *throughput*, the process by which decisions are taken and plans for administration and implementation are made concrete. It is this last category that, as she points out, remains so opaque considering its crucial importance.

As this would suggest, there is immense focus in the policy, politics, and administration literatures on the democratic qualities of input in particular. Those focused on democratic renewal have focused their energies almost exclusively in this area. Indeed, a recent 'state of the field' article describes two cultures of democratic theory—one normative, one empirical—which narrowly focus on the inputs to decision-making, in the form of votes, demands citizens and civil society actors make, and the institutions that channel and funnel these demands to legislatures (see Sabl 2015). Output, where it is considered, is seen largely as a product or consequence of input, although of course the vast literature on public administration would suggest it is rather more complicated in practice. Even so, there remains relatively little emphasis on processes of *throughput*, whose democratic credentials might be better unpacked. Schmidt's account is a call for more focus on how decisions are turned into action. The findings I develop here provide fresh insights into these processes, and how we might improve them as well. In particular, I highlight how an emphasis on enhancing the quality of input to policymaking on obesity, when it comes at the expense of throughput, can further compound the problems associated with a dullening of emotion and blunting of critique and contestation described above.

Most pertinently, my analysis highlights differences in the institutional architectures of policy debate and policy work across the two cases which help to explain Britain's slightly better performance on this dimension. Simply put, the British debate has had institutions that better enable scrutiny, debate, and contestation downstream in the policy process, after a decision has been made and as it gets turned into policy action. The point is not that such bodies have been absent in Australia and present in Britain, but that the bodies have been stronger and more effective in the latter. While ongoing expert and stakeholder bodies have existed in the Australian case, they have generally taken a long time to form together, met very infrequently, been very low profile and exclusive, and operated under strictly limited terms of reference. The expert advisory board for ANPHA, for instance, was not established until mid-2011, some 12 months after the agency first began operating and over 2 years since the legislation for its establishment was drafted. This has enabled an implementation phase in which powerful actors are able to push policy in their interests, all beyond the spotlight of publicity. In Britain, in contrast, the institutional architecture through which the obesity debate has been channelled has encouraged a messier, more recursive debate with greater potential to keep discussion on the issue bubbling along. Importantly, some innovative sites of debate have carried on continuously or periodically, at least for a time—a process which has served to remind all the actors that just because a decision has been reached that does not mean the discussion is over. The Foresight process, for instance, spawned an expert advisory body that until recently had close access to the Secretary of State and senior public servants. Perhaps more important still has been the FSA and its open board meetings. Though, as explained in the introduction, never set up with discussion of obesity policy in mind, this issue quickly became one of the key items in the board's remit, and it has been on aspects relating to obesity and nutrition that the board has done its most controversial work—so much so that it attracted considerable criticism from the food industry, ultimately resulting in a significant reduction in the FSA's powers and responsibilities.[4] Nevertheless, over most of the period of my analysis and before it, the board has been an important site of debate on obesity, in particular making high-profile pushes for traffic light labelling and firmer food reformulation targets. These continued periodically throughout the decade, providing an institutional outlet through which to put considerable scrutiny on government poli-

---

[4]See Lang (2010) for a knowledgeable insight into the neutering of the FSA's responsibilities in relation to public health.

cies around 'a comprehensive approach' (under New Labour) and 'nudge' theory (under the Coalition) respectively.

This difference between the two cases, to be clear, is in extent rather than kind. While the UK debate performs better relative to the Australian one in my analysis, this should not be read as a statement that the democratic qualities of throughput in the UK are the ideal. Certainly, any such suggestion would surprise those actually engaged in the debate. The open board meetings of the FSA and the Foresight process, and subsequent expert committee, are not prototypes. Each has significant flaws and weaknesses. Most notably, neither has been robust enough to resist or subvert pressure in recent times from the Coalition government. The expert committee has been disbanded and the authority of the FSA largely eroded (though, in fact, even these actions have served to stir controversy and garner greater public scrutiny of the actions of government and private interests). Nevertheless, combined these sites display some general features that seem crucial to generating throughput legitimacy: a critical orientation to government; access to ministers and top officials; the capacity to monitor progress; and the capacity to publicise problems or inconsistencies in the implementation of policy. Such mechanisms can play a crucial role in ensuring democratisation downstream in the policy process as well (see Boswell forthcoming).

But, again, the preceding analysis has salient lessons for a public health audience as well. Chiefly, it suggests that public health experts and advocates would be better served targeting their resources further 'downstream' in the policy process. Though advocates have had significant initial success in getting obesity onto the agenda, my analysis reveals that these actors have had considerably more difficulty effectively 'staying' with the recursive, drawn-out process of policymaking—something civil society actors notoriously struggle with (see Mazey and Richardson 2012). They cannot devote the time and resources to be on hand as their clarion calls for action subsequently filter through Parliamentary inquiries, technical task force discussions, administrative committees, and beyond into the realm of complex, networked policy implementation. Above I mark out the differences in the institutional architecture of the debates in both Australia and the UK, but I could equally point back to the last section on conciliation and conflict to suggest that aspects of advocacy practice and culture remain obstacles as well. Devoting greater energy and more resources to telling their narrative about obesity 'along' this process will allow them to better scrutinise and critique efforts to contain or neutralise the issue, working to stoke the political 'war on obesity' along more effectively.

A Final Word

I want to reiterate, as I have said all along, that the implications I have laid out in this chapter will not 'win' the war on obesity, let alone lay out a blueprint for solving other complex and contested policy issues. For policymakers and public managers, enabling affective embodiment, taking heed of evidence on emotions, structuring opportunities for conflict and conciliation to occur together, and pursuing greater throughput legitimacy will not solve the problem, either as isolated moves or as a collective effort. For public health advocates, in turn, engaging with expert citizens, developing and taking more seriously qualitative, interpretive research on the lived experience of obesity, becoming feistier about perceived injustices in governance network interactions, and devoting greater resources to advocacy downstream in the policy process will not ensure their preferred policy outcomes eventuate, either. Policymaking on wicked issues like obesity does not work like that. Neither does their politics.

The metanarrative I have developed here would suggest that the primary concern of both groups ought to be more modest yet more fundamental. They need to work to make sure that the real war on obesity, the political battle over its nature and meaning, does not peter out. Representing, claiming, contesting, and transmitting knowledge remain crucial tasks. But by making space for emotion and affect as well as experts and evidence, and enabling and structuring ongoing contestation as well as channelling moments of compromise and conciliation, it may be possible to again raise the profile of obesity as an issue of government attention. Doing so might enable public health actors to sustain stronger institutional architecture and higher political capital through which to challenge the watery, tokenistic compromises of the status quo, and follow through effectively on any new policy commitments.

The policy 'war on obesity'—as with that on drugs, on poverty, on social exclusion, on climate change—may never be won. But, as I have shown, it may very well be possible for the political war to be fought in a more sustained fashion, on a more even footing. That remains an outcome worth fighting for.

References

Banwell, C., Broom, D., Davies, A., & Dixon, J. (2013). *Weight of modernity: An intergenerational study in the rise of obesity*. New York: Springer.

Blaug, R. (2002). Engineering democracy. *Political Studies, 50*(1), 102–116.

Boswell, J. (2014). 'Hoisted with our own petard': Evidence and democratic deliberation on obesity. *Policy Sciences, 47*(4), 345–365.

Boswell, J., & Corbett, J. (2015b). Stoic democrats? Anti-politics. Elite cynicism and the policy process. *Journal of European Public Policy, 22*(10), 1388–1405.

Downs, A. (1972). Up and down with ecology: The 'issue-attention cycle'. *The Public Interest, 28*, 38–50.

Easton, D. (1965). *A systems analysis of political life*. New York: Wiley.

Gard, M., & Wright, J. (2001). *The obesity epidemic: Science, morality and ideology*. New York: Routledge.

Griggs, S., & Howarth, D. (2013). *The politics of airport expansion in the United Kingdom: Hegemony, policy and the rhetoric of 'sustainable aviation'*. Manchester: Manchester University Press.

Gutmann, A., & Thompson, D. F. (1996). *Democracy and disagreement*. Cambridge, MA: The Belknap Press.

Hendriks, C. M. (2011). *The politics of public deliberation: Citizen engagement and interest advocacy*. London: Palgrave Macmillan.

Hoppe, R. (2005). Rethinking the science–Policy nexus: From knowledge utilization and science technology studies to types of boundary arrangements. *Poiesis & Praxis, 3*(3), 199–215.

Jasanoff, S. (1990). *The fifth branch: Science advisors as policymakers*. Cambridge, MA: Harvard University Press.

Jasanoff, S. (1996). Beyond epistemology: Relativism and engagement in the politics of science. *Social Studies of Science, 26*(2), 393–418.

Kline, S. (2015). Moral panic, reflexive embodiment and teen obesity in the USA: A case study of the impact of 'weight bias'. *Young Consumers, 16*(4), 407–419.

Korinek, R., & Veit, S. (2015). Only good fences keep good neighbours! The institutionalization of Ministry-Agency relationships at the science-policy nexus in German food safety. *Public Administration, 93*(1), 103–120.

Lang, T. (2010, July 21). What a carve up: The coalition is wrong to dismember the Food Standards Agency at the time it is needed most. *The Guardian.* Retrieved January 17, 2013, from http://www.guardian.co.uk/commentis-free/2010/jul/21/fsa-what-a-carve-up

Lupton, D. (2013). *Fat.* London: Routledge.

Mansbridge, J., Bohman, J., Chambers, S., Estlund, D., Føllesdal, A., Fung, A., et al. (2010). The place of self-interest and the role of power in deliberative democracy. *Journal of Political Philosophy, 18*(1), 64–100.

Mazey, S., & Richardson, J. (2012). Environmental groups and the EC: Challenges and opportunities. In A. Jordan (Ed.), *Environmental policy and the EU: Actors, institutions and processes.* London: Earthscan.

Milewa, T., & Barry, C. (2005). Health policy and the politics of evidence. *Social Policy and Administration, 39*(5), 498–512.

Newman, J. (2012). Beyond the deliberative subject? Problems of theory, method and critique in the turn to emotion and affect. *Critical Policy Studies, 6*(4), 465–479.

Orsini, M. (2015, July 8–10). Mobilizing metaphors: Complex moral emotions and the affective politics of obesity. *10th annual conference on interpretive policy analysis.* Lille: Science Po.

Orsini, M., & Scala, F. (2006). Every virus tells a story: Toward a narrative centered approach to health policy. *Policy and Society, 25*(2), 109–130.

Rail, G., Holmes, D., & Murray, S. J. (2010). The politics of evidence on 'domestic terrorists': Obesity discourses and their effects. *Sociological Theory and Health, 8*, 259–279.

Rummens, S. (2011). Staging deliberation: The role of representative institutions in the deliberative democratic process. *Journal of Political Philosophy, 20*(1), 23–44.

Sabl, A. (2015). The two cultures of democratic theory. *Perspectives on Politics, 13*(2), 345–365.

Sanders, L. (1997). Against deliberation. *Political Theory, 25*(3), 347–376.

Schmidt, V. A. (2013). Democracy and legitimacy in the European Union revisited: Input, output and 'throughput'. *Political Studies, 6*(1), 2–22.

Thompson, S., & Hoggett, P. (Eds.). (2012). *Politics and the emotions*. London: Continuum.

Wanna, J., & Weller, P. (2003). Traditions of Australian governance. *Public Administration, 81*(1), 63–94.

Warin, M., Turner, K., Moore, V., & Davies, M. (2008). Bodies, mothers and identities: Rethinking obesity and the BMI. *Sociology of Health and Illness, 30*, 97–111.

Index

© The Editor(s) (if applicable) and The Author(s) 2016
J. Boswell, *The Real War on Obesity*,
DOI 10.1057/978-1-137-58252-2

Printed in the United States
By Bookmasters